Staying Healthy Abroad
A Global Traveler's Guide

Staying Healthy Abroad

A Global Traveler's Guide

Christopher Sanford, MD

UNIVERSITY OF WASHINGTON PRESS

Seattle

Printed and bound in the United States of America
Design by Katrina Noble
Composed in Cala, typeface designed by Dieter Hofrichter
22 21 20 19 18   5 4 3 2 1

UNIVERSITY OF WASHINGTON PRESS
www.washington.edu/uwpress

LIBRARY OF CONGRESS CATALOGING-IN-PUBLICATION DATA
Names: Sanford, Christopher, author.
Title: Staying healthy abroad : a global traveler's guide / Christopher Allen Sanford, MD.
Description: Seattle : University of Washington Press, [2018] | Includes bibliographical references and index. |
Identifiers: LCCN 2018012493 (print) | LCCN 2018026675 (ebook) | ISBN 9780295744391 (ebook) | ISBN 9780295744384 (pbk. : alk. paper)
Subjects: LCSH: Travel—Health aspects. | International travel—Health aspects. | Tourism—Health aspects.
Classification: LCC RA783.5 (ebook) | LCC RA783.5 .S263 2018 (print) | DDC 613.6/8—dc23
LC record available at https://lccn.loc.gov/2018012493

To Sallie

CONTENTS

ACKNOWLEDGMENTS

I would like to thank the following consultants: on motor vehicle safety, Drs. William Foege and Charles Mock; on men's health, Dr. Jay Keystone; on pediatrics, Dr. Sheila Mackell; on family medicine, Drs. Morhaf Al Achkar, Justin Osborn, and Adam McConnell; on travel medicine, Anne C. Terry, ARNP, and Britt Murphy, ARNP; on high-altitude medicine, Dr. Andrew Luks; on women's health, Dr. Christina Tanner; on LGBTQ travelers, Genya N. Shimkin; on dive medicine, Dr. Ed Kay; on infectious disease, Drs. Paul Pottinger and Vernon Ansdell; on otolaryngology (ear, nose, and throat) , Dr. Greg E. Davis; on disaster medicine, Drs. Susan Briggs and Helen Miller, and Darlene B. Matsuoka; on pharmacology, pharmacists Elyse Tung and Alvin Goo; on security, Chris Presley and Adam Rozelle. I would also like to thank the staff of University of Washington Press: Lorri Hagman, Margaret Sullivan, Michael O. Campbell, Mary Yang, Katrina Noble, Casey LaVela, and copy editor Heath Lynn Silberfeld, for their many valuable suggestions. I am indebted to Drs. Elaine C. Jong and Tom E. Norris, University of Washington, for their mentorship over the years. And thanks most of all to my wife, Sallie, and our sons, Nate and Henry, my favorite travel companions.

Introduction

The world is a book, and those who do not travel, read only a page.

AUGUSTINE OF HIPPO, 354–430 CE

If the Internet were everything it is cracked up to be, we would all stay home and be brilliantly witty and insightful. Yet with so much contradictory information available, there is more reason to travel than ever before: to look closer, to dig deeper, to sort the authentic from the fake; to verify, to smell, to touch, to taste, to hear.

PAUL THEROUX, *The Last Train to Zona Verde*

THE PURPOSE OF this guide is to reduce your risk of illness and injury while traveling abroad. Although the focus is on travel to low- and middle-income nations, much of this advice applies to travel in the industrialized world as well. My emphasis is on common illnesses and injuries. As titillating as shark attacks and lightning strikes may be, they are low on my list of priorities; if something occurs less frequently than one-in-a-million, it probably isn't going to happen to you. I am concerned with common problems: car crashes, travelers' diarrhea, hepatitis A.

One theme of this work is that noninfectious risks are generally underappreciated by global travelers and underemphasized by pre-travel providers. Another key theme is that these threats are not random; prudent precautions can reduce risk. Reading through travel health literature, I am struck again and again by the fact that risk is less determined by where you go than by what you do. It is just a slight overstatement to say that there are no risky destinations—only risky travelers.

And why should you travel outside high-income nations? Why should you voluntarily visit a land with sketchy plumbing and dodgy roads? The lure of these countries is difficult to explain. Those of us who gravitate toward travel in the poorer regions of the world experience equal parts adrenaline and wonder. Travel to lower-income nations will elevate the mundane into the realm of the considered; it will show you what is left of you when you remove routine and reflex.

It is important, I think, to realize that our own corner of the world is not representative; most of us who live in North America and Western Europe are, in fact, wealthy and lucky. For many of us, travel to other nations is a life-changing experience. During our travels we may come to appreciate, in a manner that would be impossible had we remained within Euro-America, the vast magnitude of global inequalities; after our return, we may newly appreciate our usual environs.

People travel the globe for myriad reasons: to study, to serve, to recreate, to conduct business, to visit the land of their forebears. Regardless of our motivation, a few precautions will minimize the risk of illness or injury during our travels; hence my guide.

Travel Medicine Q&A

Q **What do you mean by *lower-income nations*?**
A There is no perfect term. *Third World* gave way to *developing*, which in turn gave way to *low- and middle-income nations* and, most recently, to the *Global South*.

The World Bank categorizes every economy as high, middle, or low. (The per capita gross national income in middle-income countries was, in fiscal year 2018, between US$1,005 and US$12,235.) It then further subdivides economies; India, for example, is considered a lower-middle-income nation. The

United Nations favors the terms *less developed nation* and *least developed nation*.

Pew Research Center statistics indicate that only 7% of the world's population is considered high income (income over US$50/day, or US$18,250/year). High-income nations include the US and Canada, Australia, New Zealand, Japan, and South Korea, along with Western Europe. Most of the rest of the world is middle income or low income.

Q **Is *travel medicine* really a medical specialty, or did you just make that up?**

A It exists. It is a new specialty, extant for approximately forty years. It has been defined as "the discipline devoted to the maintenance of the health of international travelers through health promotion and disease prevention" (J. S. Keystone et al., eds. *Travel Medicine*, chapter 1). It is an interdisciplinary field, drawing on the fields of infectious disease, public health, preventative medicine, and a host of other medical specialties and subspecialties.

Q **Can any medical provider give me advice regarding travel medicine?**

A No. Most medical providers do not see a sufficient number of international travelers to be proficient. You want to find someone who advises international travelers on a regular basis.

Q **How do I find a pre-travel provider?**

A Both the International Society of Travel Medicine (ISTM) and the American Society of Tropical Medicine and Hygiene (ASTMH) maintain a list of travel clinics on their websites: www.istm.org, www.astmh.org. Many US universities have travel clinics; some see students only, some see anyone. Medical organizations such as health maintenance organizations (HMOs) often have travel clinics.

Q How long before our trip do we need to visit the travel clinic?

A We like a month to six weeks or longer if we can get it. Most vaccines take about one to two weeks to kick in (phrasing this more formally, the antibody response initiated by vaccines requires one to two weeks to attain protective levels).

A few vaccine series are given over four weeks. Another advantage of being seen at least a month prior to your departure is that you have time for a pre-travel trial of medications with potential for side effects, such as those that prevent malaria, while you are still in-country. However, travel clinics will see travelers at any time prior to their trip.

What This Book Is Not

This guide is not intended to replace your visit to a pre-travel provider, who will evaluate your personal health history, itinerary, and planned activities, then make specific recommendations. Rather, its ambition is to prepare you for your consultation with your pre-travel provider and equip you with strategies that will keep you fit during your travels.

Travel medicine, like other fields of medicine, is an ever-changing discipline. Recommendations are updated as new studies are incorporated into the body of knowledge on which we advisors base our advice. I have attempted to offer all prevention and treatment protocols with the latest available information, but readers should consult their own physicians for the most up-to-date recommendations. You should confirm all drug doses and discuss possible side effects and interactions with other drugs with your pre-travel provider. This is a guide, not a comprehensive medical text; discussion of many topics is necessarily summary. Readers seeking a more in-depth discussion of topics pertinent to travel medicine should look to the textbooks of travel medicine listed at the back of this guide in Resources for Global Travelers.

The field of travel medicine, encompassing as it does all illnesses and manner of injury in all nations, is too vast for any one person to master. If you have suggestions, additions, or corrections, please drop me a line at my publisher's office:

Christopher Sanford
c/o University of Washington Press
Box 359570
Seattle, WA 98195–9570 USA

Overview

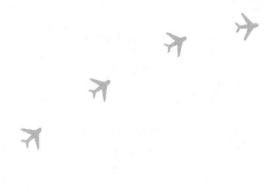

1

Planning for Healthy International Travel

The Bottom Line

Seeing a pre-travel provider can markedly reduce your odds of illness and injury while abroad. A pre-travel provider is a health professional—usually a physician, nurse practitioner, physician assistant, or nurse—with expertise in the health issues of international travelers. During the pre-travel encounter your provider will evaluate you and your itinerary, then make recommendations concerning vaccines, medications, strategies to reduce risk of accidents, and other salient topics.

The Pre-Travel Encounter

You and your pre-travel provider have a number of topics to discuss during the pre-travel encounter:

> Your past medical history
  - Medications
  - Allergies
  - Surgeries

- Hospitalizations
- Immunization history
- Prior antimalarial use
- *When applicable*: safer sex, STIs, birth control, and/or possibility of pregnancy

> Itinerary
- Where and when you're going
- Planned activities
- Type of accommodation

> Immunizations
- Which immunizations the provider advises for this trip
- Which immunizations, if you can't afford all of them, are most important

> Malaria
- Where malaria is and is not present in countries you will be visiting
- Personal protection measures (i.e., minimizing bug bites)
- Prophylactic medication options

> Travelers' diarrhea
- Dietary choices to minimize risk
- Pros and cons of antibiotic self-treatment for travelers' diarrhea

> Urban medicine
- Road traffic injury risk reduction
- Crime
- Security

> Special topics, if your itinerary so necessitates
- High-altitude illness
- Scuba diving

> Emergency medical evacuation insurance
- Travelers to low-income countries should consider purchasing evacuation insurance. Emergent medical evacuation via jet is extraordinarily pricey: about US$50,000–$100,000. A number of companies and organizations provide emergency medical evacuation insurance, such as International SOS, MedAire,

SafeTrip, and Divers Alert Network (DAN). You pay a fee up front, and if emergent evacuation is required, the company flies you to an appropriate medical facility without additional charge. The online company Squaremouth compares travel insurance products, including evacuation insurance, from every major provider in the US.

> How to contact the travel clinic when you're out of the country (usually by e-mail)
> Follow-up screening after your trip, if needed

If you have health insurance, phone the member services department prior to your departure and ask what the company covers. Some plans will cover you when you travel abroad; some will not. (Medicare, for example, does not cover people outside the US.) Sometimes those that do will require that you bring back any receipts for medical care, and they will reimburse you. Every plan is different. This is much easier to research from your country of origin prior to your trip.

US Department of State Travel Advisories

In 2018 the US Department of State replaced its former system of country-specific warnings and advisories with a four-level schema of travel advisories. Every country advisory is designated at one of four levels:

Level 1: Exercise Normal Precautions
Level 2: Exercise Increased Precaution
Level 3: Reconsider Travel
Level 4: Do Not Travel

Factors considered by the Department of State when assigning these levels include crime, terrorism, civil unrest, threats to health, natural disasters, and time-limited events such as elections or political protests.

Travelers who are US citizens should enroll in the US Department of State's Smart Traveler Enrollment Program (STEP), a free service that enrolls travelers with the nearest US embassy or consulate during their travels. This allows travelers to receive information from the embassy regarding topics pertinent to safety, and emergency information concerning natural disasters, civil unrest, or a family emergency. The process of signing up doesn't take long. See https://step.state.gov. In addition, always inform friends and family of your itinerary, and carry a mobile phone if possible in regions with cell phone reception.

Infectious Diseases

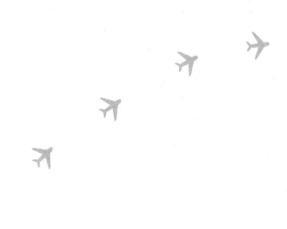

2

Immunizations

The Bottom Line

- You should be current on the usual domestic vaccines, including influenza, hepatitis A, and tetanus-diphtheria-pertussis.
- Vaccination for hepatitis B is a good idea for almost every traveler.
- Vaccination for yellow fever is recommended for travel to most countries in tropical South America and tropical Africa; for travel to many countries, it is required.
- Depending on your itinerary, duration of stay, and planned activities, other vaccines may be recommended.

IT IS CONVENIENT to view each vaccine as falling into one of two categories: routine (domestic) and travel.

Routine Immunizations

Although most people do not associate routine, or domestic, vaccines with international travel, in the big scheme of things these vaccines probably provide more protection to travelers than do vaccines recommended specifically for travel. It is prudent for the international traveler to remain current on all standard vaccines. The current schedule of recommended vaccines for adults is posted at the Centers for Disease Control (CDC) website: www.cdc.gov. Each is discussed in the following sections.

DIPHTHERIA, TETANUS, PERTUSSIS

Assuming you received the standard diphtheria, tetanus, and pertussis (DTaP) series as a child, you should get a tetanus shot every ten years. Historically, in the US, this is given as a dip-tet, or Td, which provides protection against tetanus and diphtheria. In 2005 a new combination vaccine, Tdap, was released on the US market; it covers pertussis (whooping cough) as well. Both diphtheria and pertussis are more prevalent in lower-income nations. One dose of Tdap is now routinely given to children in the US at age 11 or 12; those who did not receive it at that age should substitute Tdap for one booster dose of Td.

MEASLES, MUMPS, RUBELLA

Measles, mumps, and rubella (MMR) are far more common outside of high-income nations. Since 2010, measles cases in the US have ranged between 55 and 667 per year. In 2016 ninety thousand deaths occurred worldwide due to measles.

Those born in or after 1957 require immunization for MMR. The first dose is usually administered at about fifteen months; the second at age 4 to 6 years, although it can be given as soon as four weeks after the first.

Adult travelers with neither a history of having received two doses nor lab testing showing immunity should receive immunization for MMR. Most US colleges and universities will not allow students to enroll until they have received a second dose of MMR or demonstrate protection via a blood test. The CDC does not recommend vaccination for those born prior to 1957, as they are presumed to have immunity to these illnesses.

POLIO

Polio is not yet eradicated, although a decades-long campaign has come close to eliminating polio in most of the world. The incidence has decreased by over 99% since 1988; in 2017, there were only twenty-two cases worldwide.

For adults who received the usual four-dose childhood series (either oral or injection), a single polio booster is advised for those traveling to regions with recent or ongoing polio transmission (including, as of 2017–18, Afghanistan, Pakistan, Syrian Arab Republic [Syria], Nigeria, and Democratic Republic of the Congo [DRC]); further boosters are not necessary. (*Note:* Oral polio vaccine—"the sugar cube"—is no longer available in the US; in the US, all polio immunizations are given via injection.)

HEPATITIS A

Hepatitis A is one of the most common vaccine-preventable illnesses of travelers. It is caused by a virus that is spread by contaminated food and water. (In medical parlance, this route of spread is known by the rather unsettling term *fecal–oral transmission.*)

Hepatitis A is a relatively mild illness in children but will land an adult in bed for several weeks; in those above age 40 it carries a 2% death rate. Even in those who survive, it's not pleasant. Your skin and sclerae (the whites of your eyes) turn an alarming yellow-orange (jaundice). The discoloration of the skin is more difficult to detect in dark-skinned people, but the change in color of the sclerae is evident in everyone.

Additionally, those infected develop nausea, belly pain, sweats, and general misery. You can get it only once, but for people who've been through it, once is one time too many. The vaccine is by far the preferable option.

The hepatitis A vaccine series is simple: two shots, at least six months apart. The duration of immunity to hepatitis A following this vaccine series appears to be lifelong. Children in the US now receive this routinely, usually between the first and second birthdays.

Myths Regarding Hepatitis A

"If I choose my food and drink with caution, I'll be okay."
Hepatitis A is common outside of high-income nations, and you can't tell by looking at food and water whether they're safe or contaminated. The same strategies that may reduce your risk of travelers' diarrhea may reduce your risk of hepatitis A, but not to the point that you want to take a pass on the vaccine.

"I was born in a low-income country, so I'm probably protected."
There is some truth to this claim. Indeed, many people born in low-income countries have had this illness, most commonly during childhood, and are protected. However, given that many people are not protected, assuming that someone is protected is risky. People born in low-income countries should either:

- receive an antibody blood test to see if they have protection, and get the vaccine series if they do not, or
- simply get the vaccine series.

"It's not required, so it must not be important."
"Not required" doesn't mean "not advised." Hepatitis A is much more common in international travelers than yellow fever, for which vaccination is required to enter some countries. You should base your choice of vaccines on what diseases your travel places you at risk for, not on what is required.

"I'm leaving in less than two weeks. I've read that hepatitis A vaccine takes two weeks to kick in, so I'll get gamma globulin instead."
That used to be the recommendation, but physicians now realize that even if you get your first hepatitis A vaccine dose on the way to the airport, you'll be protected at your destination. It works like this:

After receiving the first hepatitis A immunization, your body does indeed require about two weeks to develop protective antibodies (the specific molecules that your body manufactures in response to a vaccine or infectious organism and which prevent a disease). However, hepatitis A has a minimum incubation period of two weeks, so even if you have the bad luck to be exposed to hepatitis A during your first meal abroad, a race then occurs between the incubation of the disease and the formation of antibodies. Antibodies form more quickly, so you do not get the illness.

After the first immunization for hepatitis A you are protected for at least six to twelve months. You should get the second and final shot of the series six months after the first, which extends your protection for life. (Gamma globulin, which was given for protection from hepatitis A prior to a hepatitis vaccine coming onto the US market in 1995, provides protection for only a few months.)

For maximal protection, an option for adults over age 40, immunocompromised persons, and those with chronic liver disease or other chronic medical problems, should they be departing in less than two weeks after the pre-travel consult, is to receive a single injection of gamma globulin (also called immunoglobulin [IG]) at the same time as the first dose of hepatitis A vaccine (at a different body site).

HEPATITIS B

Although more rare than hepatitis A in travelers, hepatitis B is a more serious illness, and vaccination for this disease should be considered by almost every traveler. Unlike hepatitis A, which is spread by contaminated food and water, hepatitis B is transmitted by blood and sex, and from mother to baby at birth. In addition to having more severe symptoms and lasting longer, hepatitis B often, unlike hepatitis A, develops into a lifelong carrier state, with significant risk of liver failure.

Significantly, some long-stay travelers who report no potential risks for acquiring hepatitis B (no new partners in their sex lives, no needle pokes or tattoos) do periodically acquire this disease. Possibly, the virus is entering those who lack apparent risk factors via breaks in the skin that are too small to notice. Medical or dental procedures utilizing contaminated instruments can also spread hepatitis B.

The vaccine series consists of three shots. You should receive the second and third shots one and sixth months after the first. (In vaccine lingo, you get the shots at time 0, 1, and 6 months.) Protection is lifelong; there is no need for booster shots.

A new two-dose hepatitis B vaccine, HEPLISAV-B, was approved by the FDA in 2017. The two doses are administered one month apart.

The routine use of hepatitis B vaccine in infants has been recommended in the US since 1991.

Hepatitis B Accelerated Schedules

If you cannot receive the hepatitis B series utilizing the usual schedule because your departure is less than six months away, you can employ an accelerated series schedule, during which you get three shots of hepatitis B vaccine prior to your trip (on days 0, 7, and 21 to 28), then a fourth shot one year after the first. Long-term protection is ensured by receiving the fourth and final shot. If you are receiving hepatitis A only, you do not need to use an accelerated series because one injection provides a high level of protection for at least six to twelve months.

There is also an accelerated schedule called Twinrix, consisting of four shots, given at days 0, 7, and 21, and one year. Twinrix is a combination hepatitis A and hepatitis B immunization product. Its standard schedule is three shots, at time 0, 1 month, and 6 months. Its benefits are that it's a little cheaper than getting hepatitis A and B vaccines separately, and you receive three shots as opposed to the five that you would get if you received the hepatitis A and B series separately.

INFLUENZA

Influenza, as anyone who has had it can tell you, is not just a bad cold. It is a severe illness that lands the average victim in bed for a couple of weeks. The worldwide influenza pandemic of 1918–1919 killed an estimated fifty million people; in recent decades, influenza has killed between three thousand and eighty thousand people every year in the US alone.

Travelers get influenza more frequently than do people who stay home. Additionally, travelers are more prone to acquiring it off-season. In the US, the influenza season is October to April. South of the equator (e.g., in Australia), this is exactly the opposite six months: April to October. Near the equator, there is no seasonality; influenza occurs sporadically throughout the year.

Influenza is common in international travelers; in fact, it is the most common vaccine-preventable disease in travelers. A Swiss study found that international travelers developed it at a rate of 1 case for every 100 person-months abroad. Given that flu vaccine is inexpensive and has minimal side effects, the influenza immunization should be considered for virtually every traveler, even if it is off-season in their country of origin. (However, it can be difficult to find during the off-season.)

Flu Q&A

Q **What's the difference between seasonal flu and pandemic flu?**
A Seasonal flu occurs every year.

A flu pandemic occurs when a novel influenza virus emerges for which people have minimal if any immunity. Pandemic flu spreads rapidly from person to person; assisted by jet travel, it can sweep around the world in weeks. Pandemic flu occurs infrequently (most recently in 1968–1969) and is associated with a higher-than-usual rate of illness and death.

VARICELLA (CHICKENPOX)

Chickenpox is usually a mild to moderately severe illness in children; it is often more severe in adults. If you've ever had chickenpox, you are immune for life. However, if you are not sure if you've had chickenpox, you should either receive the vaccine or get a blood test to check for immunity. (Many people who do not recall a history of chickenpox are indeed immune; they probably had cases as children so mild that the illness was not recognized as chickenpox by their parents.)

Interestingly, chickenpox has a different age distribution in different regions. In temperate countries (e.g., the US), it is primarily a pediatric illness, but in the tropics, it is primarily an illness of adults.

The usual vaccine schedule is two doses, the first at age 12 to 15 months, the second at age 4 to 6. Those above age 7 years who have not had the vaccine or the illness should receive two doses of vaccine at least four weeks apart.

If you have time for only one of the two doses prior to your departure, you will have some protection against this illness, but not as much as is provided by the full series.

PNEUMOCOCCAL DISEASE

The bacterium pneumococcus (*Streptococcus pneumoniae*) is the most common cause of community-acquired pneumonia worldwide. Risk is highest in young children, the elderly, and those with chronic medical conditions. It also causes meningitis, bacteremia (sepsis), and other infections, including middle ear infections.

Infants should receive the routine four-dose series for this. Healthy adults should receive pneumococcal conjugate vaccine (PCV13, or Prevnar 13) at age 65, followed by pneumococcal polysaccharide vaccine (PPSV23, or Pneumovax) at least one year later. Those with certain chronic medical conditions should receive immunization for PCV13 and PPSV23 prior to age 65.

SHINGLES (ZOSTER)

Shingles is a painful reactivation of chickenpox virus. Older travelers should be vaccinated for it. Zostavax was licensed by the US Food and Drug Administration (FDA) in 2006. A single dose was advised at age 60 or older. In 2017 the FDA approved a new vaccine for shingles, Shingrix, which offers a significantly higher level of protection. Zostavax provides a protection level of approximately 50%; the efficacy of Shingrix is 97% in those over age 50, 90% in those over age 70. Shingrix is administered as a two-dose series; the second dose is given two to six months after the first. The schedule for booster doses has not yet been determined. Shingrix is preferred over Zostavax; it is advised for individuals age 50 and older, and it is advised regardless of whether or not the recipient has had Zostavax, as well as regardless of whether or not the recipient has had shingles infection.

HAEMOPHILUS INFLUENZAE

Children should be current on Hib (*Haemophilus influenzae*) vaccine, which is routinely administered to infants. Children over age 5 do not need Hib vaccine unless they have certain medical conditions. One dose should be given to those older than age 5 who do not have a spleen or have a medical condition that affects spleen function, such as sickle cell anemia.

HUMAN PAPILLOMA VIRUS

Human papilloma viruses (HPVs) are transmitted by sexual contact. A majority of cases resolve without treatment, but many people with HPV develop genital warts; additionally, over 99% of cancers of the cervix are caused by HPV. Although more than thirty strains of HPV are sexually transmitted, types 6 and 11 cause 90% of genital warts, and types 16 and 18 cause 70% of cervical cancer. HPV is common: it is estimated that 80% of sexually active men and women will acquire HPV infection at some point in their lives. Most have no symptoms.

This series should be started at age 11 to 12 but can be given as early as age 9. If started before the 15th birthday, it's a two-dose series, separated by six to twelve months; if started after the 15th birthday, three doses are recommended (second dose: one to two months after the first dose; third dose: six months after the first dose). The vaccine is also indicated for young women through age 26 and young men through age 21. Initial data indicate that the vaccine offers a high level of protection.

Women who receive the vaccine should continue to receive Pap smears. No testing for HPV is recommended for men.

Standard Travel Vaccines

Depending on your anticipated itinerary, duration of stay, and planned activities, additional vaccines may be indicated.

YELLOW FEVER

Yellow fever is caused by a virus that is spread by mosquitoes. In 1793 an epidemic killed between one-tenth and one-fifth of Philadelphia's inhabitants; those who fled town included then-president George Washington. Yellow fever is now absent from North America, but it remains endemic in much of tropical South America and tropical Africa (see maps 1 and 2).

Yellow fever is serious; in some outbreaks it kills half its victims. Symptoms are jaundice (hence its moniker), nausea, vomiting, fevers, and achiness. Once someone develops yellow fever, treatment is supportive, which is physicians' buzzword for making patients as comfortable as possible and hoping they get well.

Yellow fever is quite rare in travelers from high-income countries. From 1970 to 2015, only eleven cases of yellow fever were reported in travelers—only one of whom had been vaccinated for yellow fever—from the US and Europe to West Africa (six cases) and South America (five cases).

Previously, it was recommended that travelers to regions endemic for yellow fever receive a booster dose every ten years. However, in

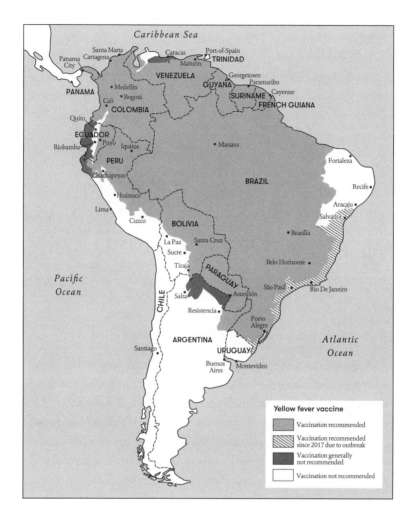

Caribbean Sea

PANAMA
Panama City
Santa Marta
Cartagena
Medellín
Cali · Bogotá
COLOMBIA
Quito
ECUADOR
Riobamba
Puyo
Iquitos
Chachapoyas
PERU
Huánuco
Lima
Cuzco
Caracas
Maturín
VENEZUELA
GUYANA
Georgetown
Paramaribo
SURINAME
FRENCH GUIANA
Cayenne
Port-of-Spain
TRINIDAD

Manaus

BRAZIL
Fortaleza
Recife
Aracaju
Salvador

BOLIVIA
La Paz
Sucre
Santa Cruz
Tiraja
PARAGUAY
Asunción
Brasília
Belo Horizonte
São Paulo
Rio De Janeiro

Pacific Ocean

CHILE
Salta
Resistencia
ARGENTINA
Santiago
URUGUAY
Buenos Aires
Montevideo
Porto Alegre

Atlantic Ocean

Yellow fever vaccine

- Vaccination recommended
- Vaccination recommended since 2017 due to outbreak
- Vaccination generally not recommended
- Vaccination not recommended

MAP 1. Distribution of yellow fever in South America
Source: Centers for Disease Control and Prevention, 2017.

2013 the World Health Organization's Strategic Advisory Group of Experts (SAGE) concluded that a single dose of yellow fever vaccine provides lifelong protection. The current recommendation is that most travelers receive one dose only, for life. If you receive a yellow fever immunization, your yellow card, under "Certificate valid from/until," should not list a specific date but instead "life of person vaccinated."

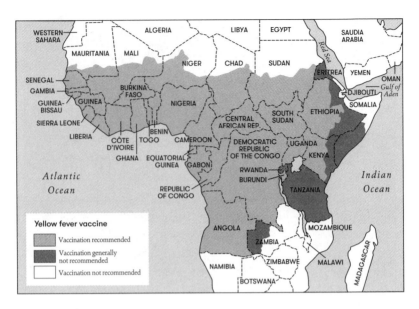

MAP 2. Distribution of yellow fever in Africa
Source: Centers for Disease Control and Prevention, 2017.

A booster is advised for some travelers, including women who were pregnant when they received their initial dose of yellow fever vaccine, and those who have received a stem cell transplant after receiving their first dose. Those infected with HIV should be revaccinated every ten years. A booster dose should be considered by those who received their previous dose more than ten years prior and will be in a higher-risk setting, based on duration of stay, season, location, and planned activities.

Many countries located in endemic regions will turn away an arrival at the airport if that traveler cannot show proof of vaccination. Additionally, many countries require evidence of yellow fever vaccination in travelers who are arriving from countries in which yellow fever is endemic, whether or not yellow fever is present in the country that the traveler is trying to enter.

A list of every nation's yellow fever requirements is available at www.cdc.gov. You should keep your vaccination record with your passport so that it is easily accessible at Customs.

Side effects from yellow fever vaccine are more common in those over age 60. Travelers over age 60 who have not received yellow fever vaccine and are going to areas with ongoing yellow fever transmission should discuss the risks and benefits of both the vaccine and the illness with their pre-travel providers. If a decision is made to forgo the vaccine, the pre-travel provider can complete the waiver section of the yellow vaccine card, which will be sufficient to get you through Customs in countries with yellow fever. It is all the more important that travelers to yellow fever–endemic areas who have not been vaccinated for yellow fever are diligent about personal protection measures (see chapter 3).

Yellow Fever Q&A

Q Who should *not* receive yellow fever vaccine?

A Pregnant women. Babies under age 9 months. People with a compromised immune system. People with thymoma (a tumor of the thymus gland) or myasthenia gravis. Those with a history of a severe allergic reaction to a prior dose of yellow fever vaccine, or any component, including egg, egg products, gelatin, or chicken protein. Also, given that WHO now states that one dose provides protection for life, anyone who has received yellow fever vaccine in the past should not have subsequent doses, unless they fall into one of the categies mentioned earlier.

Q What should I do if I have a contraindication to yellow fever vaccine and am going to an area where yellow fever is transmitted?

A One option is for your pre-travel provider to complete the "waiver" section of your immunization card, stating that you should not receive the vaccine for medical reasons. This generally suffices at Customs. However, traveling to an endemic area without the vaccine places you at risk for yellow fever. Discuss the matter with your pre-travel provider. Use of personal protection measures will reduce risk.

The only disease aside from yellow fever for which vaccination is sometimes required at international borders is meningococcal disease. One form of meningococcal disease is meningococcal meningitis, a life-threatening disease in which the meninges (the membranous coverings of the brain and spinal cord) become infected and inflamed. Signs and symptoms are fever, headache, confusion, a stiff neck, and often a rash that looks like a lot of little bruises. Although treatable with common antibiotics if rapidly diagnosed, if untreated it is fatal in more than half of the cases.

Muslims travelers making the Hajj or Umrah pilgrimage to Mecca are required to demonstrate current vaccination for meningococcal disease by the government of Saudi Arabia. This must be administered at least ten days and no more than three years prior to entry Influenza vaccine is advised but not mandatory. For additional information see https://www.saudiembassy.net/hajj-and-umrah-health -requirements.

Although it is not required, vaccination for meningococcal disease is strongly recommended for travelers to the "meningitis belt," a west-to-east stretch of land ranging across the Sahel from Senegal to Ethiopia (see map 3). Risk is particularly high during the dry season of December to June. Maps that show the area of transmission of meningococcal meningitis as a single strip across the Sahel are idealized; actually transmission occurs both within that belt and in locations scattered all around it. Travelers visiting any region in or near the meningitis belt, particularly from December through June, should consider this vaccination.

Another situation for which vaccination for this illness is advised is for those living in crowded conditions. In the US, this vaccine is advised for all college students living in dorms. Any crowded living situation (e.g., the close quarters of military recruits living in barracks) can increase the risk of transmitting this illness.

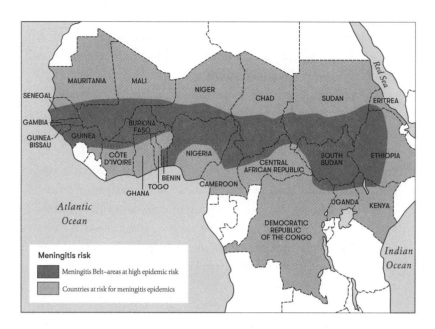

MAP 3. Distribution of meningococcal meningitis in Africa
Source: Centers for Disease Control and Prevention, 2017. *Disease data source:* World Health Organization. International Travel and Health. Geneva, Switzerland: 2012.

The CDC advises that this vaccine be routinely given to those ages 11 to 18: the first dose at age 11 or 12, the second at age 16. In the US, this is given as a quadrivalent (protective for four different serotypes) conjugate (linked to a protein) vaccine. Two quadrivalent conjugate vaccines are now available in the US: Menactra and Menveo.

For adults who have not received this vaccine before, a single dose provides protection for about five years. For those over age 7 and at ongoing risk, a booster should be given five years after the previous dose. (For those ages 9 months to 6 years, a booster is given three years after the previous dose.)

Prior to 2017, a dose of Menomune (a polysaccharide vaccine) was advised for those over age 55. In 2017, production of this vaccine was discontinued. A dose of one of the conjugate vaccines (Menactra or

Menveo) is now advised for members of this age group who are at risk. As with other vaccines, protective levels of antibodies develop about one to two weeks after vaccination.

A second type of vaccine for meningococcal meningitis, protective for serogroup B, is also available in the US. Adolescents and young adults, ages 16 to 23, may receive this. It is recommended for those with known potential exposure (e.g., a student at a college with a known outbreak of serogroup B meningococcal disease); it is also recommended for those over age 10 whose spleen has been removed or damaged, as well as those with a rare disorder of the immune system, termed *persistent complement component deficiency*. The two brands available in the US have different schedules: Bexsero is given as two doses at least one month apart; Trumenba is given as two doses at least 6 months apart.

Additional Travel Vaccines

The following vaccines are not on the standard US schedule.

TYPHOID FEVER

Typhoid fever, spread by contaminated food and water, is a disease that causes severe gastrointestinal symptoms, including severe abdominal pain, diarrhea that may be bloody (or sometimes constipation), and fever; it can be fatal.

Typhoid fever vaccine is particularly important for travelers going to higher-risk nations for a prolonged duration or planning particularly rustic travels (e.g., people staying in villages or backpacking). However, travelers should keep in mind that typhoid fever has been contracted by short-stay visitors. Risk is highest in visitors to South Asia, including India. Risk may be reduced by following the same dietary measures that reduce risk of travelers' diarrhea (see chapter 4).

Those who choose to receive this vaccine have two options: a single injection or a series of four pills; for most people, the pills are preferable. The immunization by injection consists of a single shot. The oral series consists of four pills, taken one every other day on an empty stomach until all four pills are taken. A chief benefit of the pills is that they provide protection for five years, as opposed to only two years for the injection (plus you do not get a shot, always a preferable option).

JAPANESE ENCEPHALITIS

Japanese encephalitis is caused by a virus that is spread by mosquitoes in rural South and Southeast Asia, and parts of the Western Pacific. Transmission in some countries varies by season—for example, in Vietnam the season of transmission is May to October; in Malaysia transmission is year-round. (A full listing can be found online at www .cdc.gov, under "Travelers' Health.") Most travelers do not require this vaccine; however, it should be considered by those who plan extensive travel, particularly in pig-farming or rice-farming areas. Risk is minuscule in urban areas.

Only 1 in 200 people who contract Japanese encephalitis will exhibit symptoms, but for that person it's nasty. One-third of people who become symptomatic develop neurological symptoms that fully resolve, one-third develop permanent neurological symptoms (such as paralysis), and one-third die.

The brand of vaccine approved for use in the US is IXIARO; it's given as a two-dose series, twenty-eight days apart. Minimum age is 2 months. A single booster may be given, at least one year after the primary series, for those at ongoing risk. (Different vaccines for Japanese encephalitis are used in Asia to immunize children living in endemic areas.)

Again, if you're a short-stay tourist staying in towns, you probably do not need this vaccine. If you're a wildlife biologist who will be sleeping near rice paddies, the benefits of the protection of the vaccine are probably greater than its risks. This is a vaccine to research, to discuss with your pre-travel provider, to ponder. If the vaccine were cheap, or if the disease were mild, it would be a no-brainer; but as is, it's always a tough call.

Rabies is caused by the bite, scratch, or lick of an infected mammal (e.g., dog, cat, bat, rat, monkey). In high-income nations, in which rabies is relatively rare, most cases are caused by bites of wild animals; in low-income nations, in which rabies is relatively common, most cases are caused by bites of domesticated animals (e.g., dogs).

As with Japanese encephalitis, the decision whether or not to be vaccinated for rabies can be complex. The problem is that the vaccine is expensive, and the disease is extremely rare in travelers, but when it occurs, it is extremely fatal, with a 100% mortality rate. Vaccination for rabies is not indicated for most short-duration travelers; those who should receive it include veterinarians, wildlife biologists, backpackers, those who travel to remote and isolated areas, travelers planning prolonged time abroad, and spelunkers.

The pre-exposure vaccine series consists of three shots, with one given on day 0, one on day 7, and one between days 21 to 28. This is a low-priority vaccine for short-duration travelers to common tourist destinations, such as beaches in Mexico or Thailand. Higher-risk travelers (long duration, rural travel, those with contact with wildlife, spelunkers) should receive it.

Even those who receive this vaccine require additional treatment after potential exposure to rabies. Treatment consists of two shots of rabies vaccine given three days apart. For those who do not receive the pre-exposure series, the post-exposure vaccine series is much more extensive: four shots of rabies vaccine over fourteen days (on days 0, 3, 7, and 14), plus a single shot of rabies immunoglobulin.

If bitten by an animal, you should immediately clean the wound with soap and water; this will kill a significant amount of the rabies virus should it be present (although not so much that you want to forgo post-exposure prophylaxis—injections after the bite). Whether or not you've had the pre-exposure series of rabies vaccine, you want to initiate post-exposure vaccine as soon as possible after an exposure, preferably within one to two days.

Note: None of the rabies shots—neither the series pre-exposure nor those post-exposure—is into the abdomen or particularly painful. They are simply standard shots into your upper arm. The painful injections into the abdomen haven't been given for decades.

Boosters for the primary pre-exposure series are not advised for most people. Those at elevated risk (those working with wildlife, spelunkers) should have periodic testing to ensure that their rabies antibody is at a protective level and should receive a booster dose if it is not.

CHOLERA

Prior to 2016, no vaccine for cholera was available in the US (two cholera vaccines, Dukoral and ShanChol, were available elsewhere). In 2016 the FDA approved Vaxchora, an oral cholera vaccine, for adults between ages 18 and 64 who are traveling to areas with ongoing cholera transmission.

Cholera is rare in global travelers. Between 2010 and 2014, ninety-one cases of cholera were confirmed in the US in people who traveled internationally in the week prior to illness. Of these cases, 75% were in people who had traveled to the Caribbean; 10% were in those who had traveled to India or Pakistan.

Travelers to countries endemic for cholera (including Haiti, the Dominican Republic, Yemen, and several countries in Africa) should consider this vaccine, particularly if prolonged or rural travel is anticipated. Healthcare professionals working in cholera-endemic regions should receive this vaccine.

The schedule is one dose, orally. The schedule for boosters has not yet been determined.

When a physician tells you that a vaccine gives you protection for a given disease, you should realize that protection is usually only partial. For some diseases, including hepatitis A and yellow fever, protection is excellent: Less than 1% of people, after receiving these vaccines, will develop illness after being exposed. However, some vaccines offer far less protection. Typhoid fever vaccine (both pills and the shot), for example, offers only 50% to 80% protection, which means that if you administer typhoid fever vaccine to a hundred people, then feed each of them enough typhoid bacteria to cause illness in an unvaccinated person, 20% to 50% of people will develop typhoid fever. This level of protection is better than none, so physicians recommend this for adventurous travelers, but there is room for improvement.

SMALLPOX

Smallpox has been eradicated. The last naturally occurring case occurred in Somalia in 1977. There is no need for smallpox vaccine for any traveler. The vaccine is still administered to some military personnel, and researchers working with smallpox or similar viruses. For those at ongoing risk, boosters should be given every three years.

One group of international travelers who are at particularly high risk for infectious diseases when they travel are VFRs— visiting friends and relatives: those who have immigrated to a high-income country such as the US, then return to their home in a low-income nation. There are many explanations for this increased risk; one is that VFRs may pooh-pooh the dangers of their native land and fail to see a pre-travel provider; another is that they tend to travel for longer durations. VFRs are by no means exempt from the dictum that all international travelers to low-income nations should see a pre-travel provider; indeed, given that many VFRs travel rurally and for long durations, they may benefit from pre-travel care even more than other travelers.

Vaccine Interactions

As a general rule, most vaccines can be administered at the same time.

Live viral vaccines (measles-mumps-rubella [MMR], varicella [chickenpox], zoster [shingles; Zostavax is live; Shingrix is not], intranasal influenza, yellow fever) should be given either on the same day or separated by at least twenty-eight days.

Oral typhoid vaccine is live and hence can be inactivated by some antibiotics and antimalarials, including doxycycline and Malarone. Travelers should wait at least two weeks after finishing the four capsules of oral typhoid vaccine before taking doxycycline, Malarone, or other drugs that could interfere with the typhoid vaccine. The antimalarials mefloquine (Lariam) and chloroquine (Aralen) do not decrease the effectiveness of oral typhoid vaccine. There is no interaction between the typhoid vaccine by injection, which is a killed vaccine, and oral medications.

A list of interactions among travel vaccines and drugs is at the CDC site: https://wwwnc.cdc.gov/travel/yellowbook/2018/the-pre-travel-consultation/interactions-among-travel-vaccines-and-drugs. Contraindications and precautions regarding vaccines are listed at the CDC site: https://www.cdc.gov/vaccines/hcp/acip-recs/general-recs/contraindications.html.

Vaccine Myths

"Vaccines can cause autism in children."

There is no evidence that links vaccines to autism or any other developmental or psychiatric illness. British researchers Andrew Wakefield and colleagues did publish one paper that suggested a link between measles-mumps-rubella (MMR) vaccine and autism. No one has been able to replicate their findings, which is doctor talk for "something was funny about their research." *Lancet*, the publication that published the article, has since retracted it. The following demonstrate evidence that autism and vaccines are not linked:

- The MMR vaccine was introduced in England in 1988; there was no increase in autism following this introduction.
- Autism is not more common in children who have been immunized with MMR than in those who have not.
- Autism diagnoses do not cluster around the time of MMR vaccine administration.

"I don't want to overwhelm my body's immune system by getting too many vaccines at once."

Your body can develop antibodies to hundreds of thousands, if not millions, of different antigens (molecules capable of inducing immune responses). Receiving vaccines for several diseases at once does not overwhelm your body or cause the vaccines to work less well.

"Chickenpox is always a mild illness, so why get vaccinated?"

Prior to the introduction of chickenpox vaccine in the mid-1990s, approximately eleven thousand people were hospitalized and a hundred people died from this illness each year in the US. It's mild in many kids, but some children and most adults with chickenpox are miserable for weeks; some become critically ill.

"I'm late in getting the second or third shot in a series, so I have to start over."

As a general rule, vaccines can be given late with no loss in protection once the series is completed. For example, suppose you had the first hepatitis A shot three years ago. (The usual schedule is to have two shots six to twelve months apart.) A single hepatitis A shot will provide protection for six to twelve months; protection will then wane unless the second shot is given. After the second shot is given, however, long-term immunity is just as solid as if the shots had been given exactly on schedule. In other words, once the series is complete, there is no penalty for some shots being given late.

There are two exceptions: If the oral typhoid series—usually taken as one pill every other day, four pills total—is taken over more than three weeks, the series should be repeated using the standard schedule; and if the pre-exposure rabies series (three doses, on days 0, 7, and 21 or 28) is taken over more than twenty-eight days, immunity to rabies should be assessed via a blood test.

"I have a head cold, so I can't receive vaccines."

As a general rule people with minor illnesses, such as a head cold, can still receive vaccines.

A caveat: Pregnant women, and people who are immunosuppressed, should not receive live vaccines, which include measles-mumps-rubella (MMR), oral typhoid, oral polio, intranasal flu, yellow fever, bacille Calmette-Guerin (BCG, for tuberculosis; administered to children in most of the world but not in the US), varicella (chickenpox), shingles (Zostavax is live; Shingrix is not live), rotavirus, and cholera (Vaxchora).

Vaccine Q&A

Q **What about side effects?**
A All vaccines have potential side effects. These are usually minor, such as a day or two of arm soreness. For every vaccine licensed

in the US, the CDC publishes a Vaccine Information Sheet (VIS) with a full listing of potential side effects. These are available online at https://www.cdc.gov/vaccines/hcp/vis/current-vis.html.

For example, for hepatitis A vaccine, potential side effects include soreness or redness at the site at which the vaccine is administered, low-grade fever, headache, and tiredness. Potential side effects for the measles-mumps-rubella vaccine include rash, fever, and swollen glands in the neck. Rarely, severe allergic reactions can occur.

But the key reality is that the risk from vaccines is markedly lower than the risk from the diseases from which they protect. The evidence on the benefit of vaccines is consistent and voluminous. Tetanus in the US has been reduced by more than 98%; polio is almost eliminated worldwide; smallpox, which caused an average 48,000 cases per year in the US during the twentieth century, has been eliminated from the planet. The incidence of multiple other infectious diseases, including mumps, rubella, and pertussis, has been markedly reduced in recent years—all because of vaccination.

Q **How do I prioritize, or what do I do, when the travel provider recommends more vaccines than I can afford?**

A Vaccines aren't cheap, and it's quite possible that your pre-travel provider will recommend more vaccines than you can afford. It is reasonable to ask your provider to rank these for you, in order of most to least beneficial.

Q **What if I have time to receive only a portion of a vaccine series prior to my departure?**

A In general, if you receive only a portion of a vaccine series, you will have some protection but not as much as if you had received the entire series. An exception is hepatitis A: after one dose of hepatitis A, you are fully protected for six to twelve months.

Q **I'm allergic to eggs. Are there vaccines I should avoid?**

A If your reaction to egg was life-threatening, hold off on yellow fever vaccine—see specifics below.

- *MMR (measles-mumps-rubella):* Even though eggs are used to produce MMR vaccine, it is generally safe for people with an egg allergy. However, anyone who has had a life-threatening reaction to a prior dose of MMR should avoid repeat doses.

- *Influenza:* As with the MMR vaccine, even though flu vaccine may contain a small amount of egg, it is generally safe for people with an egg allergy. Prior recommendations advised those allergic to eggs to wait in the medical office for thirty minutes after flu immunization; this is no longer advised. However, those with a history of a severe allergic reaction to a prior flu vaccine should not be vaccinated for flu again.

- *Yellow fever:* Travelers with a history of a life-threatening allergic reaction to eggs should not receive yellow fever vaccine. Those with a history of minor reactions (e.g., hives, nausea) to eggs or other vaccine components should consider skin testing prior to immunization to check for reactivity. Those who wish to receive this vaccine but have had a life-threatening reaction to eggs should consider asking their primary care provider for a referral to an allergist for consideration of desensitization therapy.

Malaria

The Bottom Line

- Malaria is a life-threatening disease. It remains a threat throughout the tropics; in 2015 it killed an estimated 429,000 people, most of them children under age 5 in sub-Saharan Africa.
- The two key components of avoiding malaria are personal protection measures (i.e., avoiding mosquito bites) and taking a preventative medication.

MALARIA IS A phenomenally unpleasant disease. Those with malaria develop extremely high fevers, they perspire to the extent that they are lying in puddles of sweat, and they shake as though stuck to an electric fence. Although I am a proponent of returning home with travel stories, no tale is worth the suffering that malaria causes. In addition, if you die it will not be you but your next of kin who will be telling the story, which is, from your point of view, a suboptimal situation.

A key aspect of malaria is that it is spread by mosquitoes; if you're not bitten by a mosquito, your risk of contracting malaria plummets. Hence the first topic to discuss is not drugs to prevent malaria but strategies by which to avoid bug bites.

Insect Avoidance Measures

Minimizing mosquito bites is fully as important as taking a proper medication. Some authorities state that it's more important.

The best two insect repellents are DEET (20%–50%) and picaridin (20%). Reapply DEET every six to eight hours and picaridin every four to six hours. A plateau effect occurs at about 50% DEET, such that higher concentrations provide minimal added protection. In addition, high concentrations of DEET can dissolve plastic.

An advantage of DEET over picaridin is that an application is effective for a longer duration (DEET: 6–13 hours vs. picaridin: 5 hours). An advantage of picaridin over DEET is that picaridin lacks DEET's petrochemical odor. These are effective at reducing bites from most insects, including mosquitoes, but they are less effective at reducing risk of tsetse fly and spider bites, and bee stings. DEET is available in the US at concentrations up to 100%; in Canada the maximum available concentration is 30%.

Two other repellent options are oil of lemon eucalyptus (OLE) (or its synthetic derivative, PMD) and IR3535. These are effective but for shorter durations than DEET. IR3535 should not be used in areas with malaria because it does not adequately repel malaria's mosquito vector.

A variety of botanical insect repellents are on the market, including citronella oil, clove oil, and lemongrass oil. These tend to be less effective and to repel insects for shorter durations than repellents such as DEET and picaridin. The best botanical is oil of lemon eucalyptus.

Repellents should be applied to exposed skin only—not beneath clothes, not onto clothes. They should not be used on cuts, wounds, or irritated skin. Damaged skin can allow increased absorption, which can potentially lead to a higher risk of toxicity. When using sprays, don't spray directly on the face; spray onto the hands, then apply to the face.

Most repellents can be used on children older than 2 months, but OLE should be used only on those over age 3.

PERMETHRIN APPLIED TO CLOTHES

Permethrin is great stuff. A synthetic chemical related to pyrethrum, found in the chrysanthemum, permethrin is cheap and doesn't leave a smell. Bugs touch it, and they drop dead.

Unlike DEET, permethrin is applied to your clothes. It comes in two forms: as a solution that you dip clothing into or as a liquid in a spray bottle. You should put permethrin on all your outer clothes: pants, shirt, socks, hat, bandana. You can even put it on delicate fabrics such as rayon, silk, and nylon.

Apply permethrin to clothing while you are not wearing it. Do so in a well-ventilated area. One application will give benefit for six weeks or six washings.

Some companies, including ExOfficio and L.L. Bean, sell clothing that is pre-impregnated with permethrin. Such clothing is effective for a specified number of washings.

In a study in Alaska, subjects who applied DEET to their exposed skin and wore permethrin-treated clothes saw more than a 99.9% reduction in bug bites; they were bitten once per hour. Subjects in another group, who used neither DEET nor permethrin, were bitten by insects an average of 1,188 times per hour, which tells us the following:

- The combination of DEET and permethrin creates a formidable barrier to insects.
- Never volunteer for a study on insect repellents.

BED NET

Sleeping under a bed net—ideally one treated with permethrin—will markedly reduce bites by insects, including mosquitoes. Additionally, it will keep all nocturnal creepy-crawlies off you. There is nothing so disconcerting as waking up at night in the jungle when something scampers across your face.

Many accommodations in regions endemic for malaria provide bed nets; lightweight nets can be purchased by travelers. Using a bed net is less important if sleeping quarters are air conditioned.

PERMETHRIN TESTIMONIAL

In 2001, I volunteered at a remote jungle clinic in the Peruvian Amazon, about fifty miles downriver from Iquitos. Although I've always used DEET, this was my first trip during which I used permethrin, and I found that I was bitten *significantly* less than during any prior trip to buggy environs.

CLOTHING

Wearing long pants and long-sleeved shirts will reduce your risk of insect-transmitted diseases, including malaria.

AVOID BEING OUTDOORS AT NIGHT

The mosquitoes that transmit malaria (genus *Anopheles*) bite at night; thus minimizing your time outdoors at night will reduce your risk of *Anopheles* mosquito bites.

HABITAT AVOIDANCE

Mosquitoes like stagnant water. If you're camping, set up your tent in a high, dry, open area, away from rivers and other bodies of water.

Insect Avoidance Measures Q&A

Q DEET stinks. And it dissolves plastic! What is it doing to my chromosomes?

A Despite DEET's vaguely carcinogenic odor, it is not a carcinogen. DEET entered the civilian market in 1957; currently, worldwide, over two hundred million people use DEET every year. If it did something funky to our chromosomes, we'd probably know about it by now.

Q What about ultrasound devices? I've seen ads that say these gizmos imitate the sounds of bats or dragonflies and frighten away the mosquitoes. And what about electronic buzzers and vitamin B1 (thiamine)?

A They don't work.

Q Ernest Hemingway wrote that when he was hunting in Africa, tobacco smoke would keep the bugs away. Does that work?

A Tobacco smoke doesn't keep bugs away. Additionally, as Hemingway noted, his technique works only if you're downwind from the game. If you're upwind, you have a more pressing concern: the game will smell *you*. Thus, if you're utilizing the Hemingway technique and the wind changes, you may experience a reversal of the hunter–prey relationship that you initially envisaged.

Antimalarials

The second key component of malaria avoidance is taking an appropriate antimalarial drug. Every year approximately 1,700 US citizens develop malaria; almost 100% of these people were not taking a preventative medicine or were taking an inappropriate drug.

It is helpful to think of malaria as falling into one of two categories: chloroquine-sensitive and chloroquine-resistant.

CHLOROQUINE-SENSITIVE MALARIA

Chloroquine remains effective in preventing malaria in only a handful of the approximately one hundred countries with malaria. (The trade name in the US for chloroquine is Aralen; trade names outside the US include Resochin, Avloclor, and Nivaquine.) Chloroquine-sensitive locations include the following:

Mexico
Countries in Central America: Guatemala, Belize, El Salvador, Honduras, Nicaragua, Panama (except Panama to the east of the Panama Canal, where malaria is chloroquine-resistant)
The island of Hispaniola (Haiti and Dominican Republic)
Some provinces of South and North Korea

Another option for chloroquine-sensitive areas is hydroxychloroquine (Plaquenil), a near-identical drug. The prices of chloroquine and hydroxychloroquine have been volatile in the US in recent years. I prescribe whichever one is cheaper.

Chloroquine is taken one time per week. You start one to two weeks before entry into the area with malaria, take it once per week while there and then for four weeks after you exit the malaria area. The adult dose is 500 mg per week.

Similarly, hydroxychloroquine is taken once per week. You start one to two weeks before entry into the area with malaria, you take it once per week while there and for four weeks after you exit the malaria area. The adult dose is 400 mg per week.

Chloroquine and hydroxychloroquine have rare side effects. Most people who take these drugs have none. The rare side effects include rash, stomach upset, and mood changes. In addition, chloroquine may exacerbate psoriasis.

In all countries with malaria other than those listed in the previous section, malaria is resistant to chloroquine. The CDC recommends that you take one of three drugs while in areas with chloroquine-resistant malaria. Each of the three is highly effective at preventing malaria. Each has pros and cons; your choice will depend on the duration of your stay, your pocketbook, and strategies to minimize side effects.

Doxycycline

Doxycycline is an underutilized and underappreciated drug for the prevention of chloroquine-resistant malaria. It's relatively cheap, and most people experience no side effects. Particularly for long-stay travelers or those on a tight budget, it's often the best choice.

Doxycycline is taken once per day. You begin one to two days prior to arrival in the malaria area, you continue taking it once per day while there, and you take it for twenty-eight days after leaving the malaria area. The adult dose is 100 mg once per day. You should not take doxycycline if you are under age 8, pregnant, or a sexually active woman of childbearing years and not using birth control.

The most common possible side effects of doxycycline are stomach upset and photosensitivity (light sensitivity). A small number of people who take doxycycline will find that the sun causes a rash. This side effect used to be thought of as fairly common; recent studies show that less than 1% of people who take doxycycline for malaria prevention develop this reaction. One reason that people who take doxycycline for malaria prevention see a low rate of photosensitivity is that they take only 100 mg per day, which is half the dose taken for certain infections, such as urethritis. Given this possibility and the low cost of doxycycline, consider asking your pre-travel provider to write for a few—say three—extra pills. Prior to your trip, take a pill once per day for three days and either get some natural sun or spend ten minutes in a tanning parlor; if nothing untoward happens to your skin, doxycycline is unlikely to make you sun sensitive when you take it for a longer duration.

Doxycycline increases the likelihood of vaginal yeast infections; women taking doxycycline may want to travel with treatment for that. Another potential side effect is esophageal ulceration. Doxycycline should not be swallowed "dry" but, rather, with a generous volume of liquid. If this pill gets stuck partway down your esophagus, it can cause an esophageal ulceration, which is a serious complication that may necessitate ending your trip and flying to a high-income nation for treatment.

A benefit of taking doxycycline for malaria is that if you are engaged in a freshwater sport such as kayaking, doxycycline will simultaneously prevent you from getting leptospirosis, a disease not uncommonly transmitted by contact with fresh water (see the section on leptospirosis in chapter 5).

Of the two forms of doxycycline, monohydrate and hyclate, monohydrate may have lower risk of GI upset relative to hyclate. However, the monohydrate form may be less effective in those who are taking acid-suppression therapy, such as cimetidine (Tagamet), ranitidine (Zantac), famotidine (Pepcid), or omeprazole (Prilosec).

RESEARCHING DRUG PRICES

It is worth taking the time to compare drug prices before buying. At the time this book was written, a helpful website at which to compare prices—both between drugs and at different pharmacies— was Good Rx: goodrx.com.

Malarone

Released onto the US drug market in 2000, Malarone is the newest of the three drugs recommended by the CDC for prevention of chloroquine-resistant malaria. Malarone, a combination of the drugs atovaquone and proguanil, is taken daily. It has the lowest risk of side effects of the three options in chloroquine-resistant areas; unfortunately, it's also the priciest of the three. The price has come down significantly since Glaxo Wellcome's patent on it expired in 2013, and it has become available as a generic.

Malarone is taken once per day. You start it one to two days before arriving in the malaria area, take it once per day while there, and continue taking it once per day for seven days after leaving the malaria area. (This is more convenient than taking doxycycline or mefloquine, each of which is taken for four weeks after leaving the malaria area [doxycycline daily, mefloquine weekly].) For adults, Malarone comes as a fixed combination tablet of 250 mg atovaquone and 100 mg proguanil.

Malarone's claim to fame is its favorable side-effect profile. You can get a rash, or stomach upset, or even psychiatric side effects from Malarone, but these are rare. Most people have no side effects at all.

Mefloquine

If mefloquine (formerly sold under the brand name Lariam) were a top-forty pop song, it would be said to be bubbling under: still on the charts but drifting downward. It remains a good drug for many people, but due to a significant rate of neurological and psychiatric side effects, its popularity is on the wane.

A single 250 mg tablet is taken by adults once per week. You should start at least two weeks before arriving at the malaria area, then take it once per week while there, and continue for four weeks after leaving the malaria area.

Potential side effects of mefloquine include vivid dreams or nightmares, anxiety, depression, and (rarely) psychosis. Of course, it also carries risk for those side effects that most drugs have: rash and GI upset.

Mefloquine can interact with multiple medications. It can lower the drug level of many common anticonvulsants, including valproic acid, carbamazepine, phenobarbital, and phenytoin; it should not be taken with any of these medications.

In 2013 the US Food and Drug Administration (FDA) added a boxed warning (sometimes known as a black box warning) to mefloquine's drug label, alerting medical practitioners and patients to mefloquine's neurologic and psychiatric side effects. Neurologic side effects, which can be permanent, include dizziness, loss of balance, and ringing in the ears.

Mefloquine-resistant malaria is present in many areas in Southeast Asia, including the Thai–Burma (Myanmar) and Thai–Cambodia borders, the western provinces of Cambodia, the Burma–China border, the Laos–Burma border, and southern Vietnam. Travelers to Southeast Asia, including Thailand, Cambodia, Burma, Vietnam, Laos, and southeast China, should use either Malarone or doxycycline for malaria prophylaxis.

WHO SHOULD AVOID MEFLOQUINE?

- Anyone who has ever had any sort of mood disorder, such as depression or anxiety, as those people have an increased risk of neuropsychiatric side effects, including exacerbating depression and anxiety. Even if your most recent episode of depression took place a while back, stay away from mefloquine.
- Travelers to regions in Southeast Asia in which malaria is resistant to mefloquine.
- Anyone with a history of cardiac conduction defects (heart block).
- Anyone with any history of seizures (aside from uncomplicated febrile seizures as a child), as mefloquine lowers the seizure threshold—that is, it makes seizure more likely.
- Anyone who has had an adverse reaction to mefloquine in the past.
- Anyone who doesn't want to take it.

Note: If you're traveling with small children, store your antimalarial medication on a high shelf, in a childproof container. Consuming even a small number of pills of antimalarial medication can cause severe illness or death in children.

In the US, antimalarials are available by prescription only. In 2017, Malarone (atovaquone and proguanil hydrochloride) became available over the counter in the UK: Adults over age 18 who weigh more than 88 pounds (40 kilograms) can purchase up to 93 tablets (for twelve weeks of travel) after discussion with a pharmacist.

Antimalarial Drugs Q&A

Q How do I determine if malaria is transmitted in a given country?

A The CDC has a very handy table online, "Yellow Fever and Malaria Information by Country" (in Chapter 3: Infectious Diseases Related to Travel, in the Yellow Book, www.cdc.gov /travel/page/yellowbook-home). This table lists, for every country in the world, if malaria is present or not, antimalarial resistance, estimated relative risk of malaria to US travelers (high, moderate, low, or very low), and recommended options for preventative medications. This table also lists yellow fever requirements and recommendations.

Q With all those side effects, should anyone take mefloquine?

A Most people who take mefloquine have no side effects. If you've taken it before and done well on it, the odds that it'll do something nasty are low, and it would be reasonable to try it again. (I take mefloquine when I'm in areas with chloroquine-resistant malaria, and I've never had any side effects. My friends have made a number of small remarks as to why I don't notice its crazy-making side effects.)

Q After what I've heard about mefloquine, there is no way I'm taking it. Should I just avoid malaria drugs altogether?

A No. Two other perfectly good drugs—doxycycline and Malarone—are available for the prevention of chloroquine-resistant malaria. Take one of those.

Q Every time I take mefloquine, I get vivid dreams. I kind of like them. Should I stop taking mefloquine?

A No. Some people enjoy the vivid dreams they have while taking mefloquine, and refer to the night after the day on which they take the mefloquine, when dreams tend to be particularly vivid, as "movie night." As long as you're not developing side effects that you do not like, such as nightmares or anxiety, there is no problem in continuing to take mefloquine.

Q I'm going to be in an area with chloroquine-resistant malaria for a long time—two years. I'm taking doxycycline because it's the cheapest. Can I really take it for two years? Should I take a break now and then?

A Yes, you can and should take it for two years. In the US, physicians routinely prescribe doxycycline (or a closely related drug, minocycline) to adolescents for acne for several years, and most develop no side effects. And no, taking a break is a very bad idea. Malaria can be a life-threatening illness, and it does your body no good to take the occasional break from the drug.

Those taking chloroquine or hydroxychloroquine daily for over five years for conditions such as rheumatoid arthritis should undergo annual retina exams to look for side effects of these medications. However, at the lower, weekly doses at which one takes these two medications for malaria, these exams are not necessary.

Q We're going to an area with malaria for our honeymoon. Which of these drugs is least risky for me to get pregnant on?

A Of the three drugs used to prevent chloroquine-resistant malaria, only mefloquine has been approved for use in all three trimesters.

Q Maybe, since I'm pregnant, I should skip the antimalarial?

A No! Malaria is a life-threatening illness, and furthermore, pregnant women and their fetuses do particularly poorly when they get malaria.

Q We really want to try to get pregnant on our honeymoon, and our hearts are set on a tropical destination—and we'd like to avoid antimalarial medications. What should we do?

A No problem. Plenty of tropical islands—Hawaii, the Bahamas, Fiji, and French Polynesia including Tahiti, among others—are free of malaria. Consider going to one of those.

Q I've heard that medications are much cheaper abroad than in the US. Is there a problem with just buying the malaria medication once I arrive?

A Potentially, yes. Quality control of pharmaceuticals in low-income nations can be spotty, and a significant number of placebo pills (pills containing sugar or some other chemical without pharmacological action) are sold in pharmacies. One study showed that as many as one pill in three sold in pharmacies in low-income nations, among more expensive drugs, was adulterated, postdated, or bogus. Another recent study found that at least twelve counterfeit preparations of artesunate, a medication used to treat malaria, were on the market in Southeast Asia. Given that malaria is a life-threatening illness, the best course is to buy malaria medications from a known and trusted source.

Q You're saying that the dosing schedule for each drug includes taking it for some time after I leave the malaria area?

A Yes. Chloroquine, Plaquenil, mefloquine, and doxycycline are taken for four weeks after exiting the malaria area, and Malarone is taken for one week after exiting the malaria area. The reason ties into the life cycle of the malaria parasite.

Suppose you are taking an appropriate drug for malaria prevention, and you are bitten by a mosquito that is transmitting malaria. The mosquito injects the malaria parasite (a one-celled protozoan organism of the genus *Plasmodium*) into your bloodstream—the drug doesn't stop that. The malaria parasite rapidly travels to your liver—the drug doesn't stop that. The malaria parasite multiplies in your liver—the drug doesn't stop that (except Malarone, which does kill the liver stage of the parasite).

Q **Wait a minute. The parasite multiplies in my liver even if I'm taking the right drug? Don't I feel sick at this point?**

A No. You feel fine. Then the malaria parasite leaves your liver and starts to multiply in your bloodstream. This is when you would start to feel sick if you are not taking an antimalarial. and this is when the drug works. The malaria parasite, after it exits your liver, is prevented from multiplying. You continue to feel fine and are not aware that it's been in your liver or elsewhere.

Q **I was born and raised in an area with year-round malaria transmission. I'm immune, right?**

A It is true that those who survive childhood in areas with year-round malaria transmission will develop semi-immunity. Infection in a nonimmune person causes misery for weeks or is fatal; malaria infection in those with semi-immunity is much milder, akin to a bad cold. However, a key point regarding semi-immunity to malaria is that if a person with semi-immunity leaves the malaria area for even a year or two, that partial protection disappears, and malaria is again a life-threatening infection. There are numerous accounts of people born and raised in equatorial Africa who then attend school in the UK or US, only to be killed by their first bout of malaria when they return to their nation of birth.

Q **What is terminal prophylaxis?**

A Infection with two of the four types of malaria, *P. vivax* and *P. ovale*, can lead to relapses years after the initial exposure. For travelers who have had prolonged exposure in malaria-endemic areas (such as Peace Corps volunteers or missionaries), terminal prophylaxis, also known as presumptive anti-relapse therapy or "the chaser," is sometimes advised to reduce the risk of relapse. This entails taking the drug primaquine for fourteen days (30 mg of base once/day for adults).

Important: Anyone who plans on taking primaquine must first be screened for G6PD deficiency, an enzyme deficiency that is particularly common among those of African, Middle Eastern, and Southeast Asian descent. Regardless of race, all people must be screened for this condition prior to taking primaquine. People with G6PD deficiency who take primaquine can develop life-threatening hemolysis (bursting of red blood cells). Only people with a normal G6PD level can take primaquine.

For those who take chloroquine, Plaquenil, doxycycline, or mefloquine for malaria prophylaxis, the fourteen days of primaquine can be taken during the final two weeks of the four weeks of the post-exposure prophylaxis, or immediately after. For those who take Malarone (atovaquone/proguanil), the fourteen days of primaquine can be taken for the seven days of post-exposure prophylaxis and for one week thereafter, or for the two weeks immediately following the one week of post-exposure prophylaxis.

THE CARRY-ALONG STRATEGY
AKA PRESUMPTIVE SELF-TREATMENT OF MALARIA
AKA STANDBY EMERGENCY SELF-TREATMENT (SBET)

This is a controversial strategy. I have strong opinions, which I will share. The rationale for carry-along drugs for malaria goes something like this: The drugs have side effects, and most people do not get malaria. Isn't it wiser to take nothing beforehand, then take a curative medication if malaria occurs?

In a word, *no*. The strongest argument against the carry-along strategy is that without a medical laboratory and a trained technician, you cannot tell if you have malaria or not. Suppose you're in the jungles of Papua New Guinea and you develop high fevers and achy joints. Do you have malaria? Maybe. Do you have dengue fever? Maybe. Do you have influenza? Maybe. Do you have something else? Maybe. You cannot tell if you or anyone else has malaria or not by the symptoms. Without laboratory tests, even a physician who specializes in tropical medicine, after a detailed history and a full physical exam, cannot tell if someone does or does not have malaria.

Swiss and German studies have shown a fourfold to tenfold increase in travelers' use (i.e., overuse) of presumptive self-treatment for malaria. Putting this differently, of those travelers who took the self-treatment medicine for presumed malaria, only 10% to 25% actually had malaria. In 2006, the *Journal of the American Medical Association* published an overview of malaria prevention in long-term travelers which concluded that self-diagnosis of malaria is likely to be incorrect.

So the whole concept of *when I get malaria I'll just do such-and-so* is flawed because when you get a fever and chills, you don't know whether or not you have malaria. Some illnesses that cause fever are minor; some are life threatening. Additionally, the malaria treatment regimens themselves have high rates of side effects, and you don't want to expose yourself to the side effects if you do not have malaria. However, the carry-along strategy continues to be utilized by some travelers, and you will no doubt come across travelers who will tell you that you're a fool to take a toxic medication for your entire stay in a malaria area. As I say, the strategy remains controversial.

Situations for which you might consider packing medications for treatment of malaria, in addition to taking it prophylactically, would be if you are extremely remote geographically—that is, if it would take you a long time to reach medical care should you fall ill, or if you are traveling for an extended duration. Always consult with your pre-travel provider should this be your plan. Travelers who develop symptoms potentially consistent with malaria should immediately seek medical care.

Currently there are several commercial diagnostic kits (e.g., BinaxNOW Malaria) that can diagnose malaria with a drop of blood obtained by fingerstick. However, these tests have not been approved for use outside of medical laboratories.

Travelers to regions where erroneous (false positive) tests for malaria are common (e.g., Africa) should continue to take a preventive medication for malaria even after receiving a diagnosis of malaria.

Malaria Q&A

Q **Is malaria in tourists rare?**

A No. Every year approximately thirty thousand residents of industrialized nations contract malaria while traveling. The CDC states that between 2004 and 2014, more than seventeen thousand Americans were infected with malaria, mostly acquired while traveling in Africa. The great majority of them were taking the wrong medication for the prevention of malaria or no medication at all.

Q **Are there any other preventive measures that long-term visitors can undertake?**

A Putting screens on windows and eliminating pools of standing water in which mosquitoes can breed (e.g., flowerpots) in the vicinity of your dwelling will reduce risk.

During travel, keep medications in the containers in which they were dispensed at the pharmacy (with the name of the medication, your name, the doctor's name, and the name of the pharmacy) Do not put the pills in an envelope, plastic bag, or other informal container. Loose, unlabeled pills, particularly in large volumes, can draw unwelcome scrutiny at Customs.

Q **Should I take a preventive medication only during the rainy season?**

A Although it's true that some countries (e.g., Botswana and Namibia) have both high- and low-transmission seasons, risk persists during the low-transmission season. Additionally, unusual weather patterns can vary the usual pattern. As a general rule, travelers should not discontinue their preventive antimalarial medication during the off season.

Q **I've heard that qinghaosu from China is a good antimalarial. Can I use that for malaria prevention?**

A Qinghaosu (more commonly known in the Western world as artemisinin) is in fact the most powerful antimalarial drug known to man. Derived from the shrub *Artemisia annua*, qinghaosu has been used by Chinese herbalists to treat malaria and other illnesses for more than a thousand years. Due to the poor bioavailability of artemisinin, semi-synthetic derivatives have been developed, including artemether and artesunate. However, the half-life of these drugs (the duration they remain in the bloodstream) is too brief to work as effective preventive medications; they are only employed for the treatment of malaria. They are best taken in combination with another drug, such as lumefantrine.

Q Another traveler at my hostel said that the medication I'm taking for malaria is poison.

A Other travelers, although well-meaning, are often misinformed. I suggest that you get your medical advice from healthcare professionals and high-quality resources (e.g., the CDC [Centers for Disease Control and Prevention], WHO [World Health Organization]).

Q I take minocycline (or doxycycline) daily for acne (or another condition). I'm going to an area for which an antimalarial is advised. What should I do?

A If you're on doxycycline 100 mg once per day, stay on it. If you're on minocycline, change to doxycycline 100 mg once per day for the duration advised for malaria (start one to two days before arrival, once per day during your time there, and once per day for twenty-eight days after leaving), then switch back to minocycline. Doxycycline is effective in both chloroquine-sensitive and chloroquine-resistant areas.

Q Do any other antibiotics protect against malaria?

A Some offer partial protection, but none offer sufficient protection, other than those mentioned above.

Q Can't I just be vaccinated for malaria?

A An effective vaccine for malaria does not yet exist. Although promising reports on new malaria vaccines are published regularly, it will probably be many years until an effective vaccine hits the market.

Q I want to donate blood. Are there any restrictions after travel?

A Per FDA guidelines, most travelers to any region with malaria cannot donate blood for one year after return. Former residents of malaria-endemic nations are deferred for three years.

Q I take nutritional and/or herbal supplements. Can these interact with my antimalarial medication?

A Yes. Ginseng, hypericum (St. John's wort), and grapefruit extract, among other supplements, can interact with chloroquine, mefloquine, and some antibiotics, including azithromycin. Inform your pre-travel provider and/or pharmacist about any supplements that you take.

Q I hear a lot about growing resistance to antibiotics. Is this an issue with antimalarial medications?

A Indeed it is. Chloroquine used to prevent malaria worldwide; now it only works in a few countries. There's growing mefloquine resistance in Southeast Asia. Malarone and doxycycline remain effective around the world—but that won't last forever.

Travelers' Diarrhea

The Bottom Line

- Travelers' diarrhea is by far the most common ailment of international travelers.
- A short course of antibiotics, begun at the onset of symptoms, can markedly shorten its duration—but antibiotics have potential side effects.

DIARRHEA IS THE scourge of travelers: As many as half of us who travel to a low-income nation will get it. Acquired by eating contaminated food and/or drink—and possibly by touching contaminated surfaces then touching your fingers to your mouth—travelers' diarrhea usually resolves without treatment but can significantly cramp your style for a few days. I'll describe a few strategies in this chapter that may reduce risk and will recommend carry-along medications that markedly lessen duration once it develops.

The great majority of travelers' diarrhea (80%–90%) is caused by bacteria, the most common of which is enterotoxigenic E. coli (ETEC). (This is not the same type of E. coli that contaminates meat and other food products, causing life-threatening illness.) Shigella, Salmonella, and Campylobacter are other bacterial causes of travelers' diarrhea; these cause a more severe form, often with fever and bloody stools. Fortunately, these are more rare in international travelers than ETEC.

Definition of Travelers' Diarrhea

An expert panel supported by the International Society of Travel Medicine (ISTM) published new definitions and recommendations for prevention and treatment of travelers' diarrhea in 2017 in the *Journal of Travel Medicine.* Prior definitions of levels of severity involved counting the number of stools passed in a twenty-four-hour period; the new definitions are based on functional impact.

Mild: Tolerable, not distressing, does not interfere with planned activities.

Moderate: distressing, or interferes with planned activities.

Severe: incapacitating, or completely prevents planned activities. May include passage of bloody stools.

Persistent: lasting over two weeks.

Travelers' Diarrhea: Risk Reduction

FOOD CHOICE

For other topics in this book I feel I'm on solid research-based ground. People who take appropriate antimalarials only very rarely develop malaria; vaccines markedly reduce risk of multiple infectious diseases. However, evidence supporting the benefit of following safe food practices for preventing travelers' diarrhea is scanty. The standard line is "Peel it, cook it, boil it, or forget it." Indeed, this very well may reduce your risk. However, people like me want to see studies—ideally a large number of studies—that show "safe eaters" experience a markedly lower rate of diarrhea than do "adventurous eaters." These studies have been done, and most of them show no difference between those who follow standard precautions and those who do not. Occasionally a study will come out that shows a slight difference; then again, at least one study showed that those staying in five-star hotels had a higher risk than those residing at less expensive accommodations. The take-home message is that the benefit of safe eating—if there is a benefit—is modest.

Despite the fact that studies do not show much benefit to eating cautiously, I still think it's prudent to follow a few basic rules.

THE BAD LIST: CULINARY NO-NOS

- *Food from street vendors*—Stands on the street—which have no refrigeration and may be using contaminated water for all cooking—are to be avoided. Food sits out for hours or days at such places, and risk of food poisoning is high. An exception might be something that's piping hot. For example, an ear of corn just off a fire should be okay. But in general, take a pass on food from street vendors.
- *Salads*—It is nearly impossible to sterilize lettuce. Often, in low-income countries, wastewater—that is, raw sewage—is used as fertilizer. Vegetables thrive on it, but it often carries Salmonella, Shigella, and a host of other pathogens. I advise limiting your salad eating to the high-income nations. If your trip is prolonged, you might consider taking a once-a-day multivitamin.
- *Raw meat or fish*—such as sushi, sashimi, or steak tartare
- *Buffets*—even at high-end hotels or restaurants, in which food sits out for several hours
- *Tap water*—even to brush your teeth (despite the fact that most cases of travelers' diarrhea are transmitted by food, not water)
- *Unpasteurized milk or other dairy products*
- *Ice*—Freezing doesn't kill most of the germs that can give you the runs.

- *Dry foods,* such as bread
- *Packaged foods*
- *Well-cooked food*
- *Boiled water*
- *Bottled water* (sealed)
- *Carbonated drinks,* such as beer and pop/soda
- *Fruits with skin, rind, or peel that you throw away,* such as banana or orange

Interestingly, although studies fail to demonstrate benefit from cautious food selection, multiple studies do show significant reduction in risk of travelers' diarrhea in those who wash their hands regularly with either soap and water or hand sanitizer gel (containing at least 60% alcohol).

Note: If you're on a cruise ship, use soap and water, not hand sanitizer gel, to reduce risk of norovirus. Norovirus isn't killed by hand sanitizer gel.

Studies show that someone eating at a different restaurant every night in a low-income nation will get diarrhea at a more frequent rate than will someone who is staying at a home and primarily eating home-cooked food. Combining this with the partial resistance to travelers' diarrhea that is seen in long-term visitors to low-income nations, those spending extended durations with families in a low-income nation will develop travelers' diarrhea at a lower rate, in episodes per time, than will a short-stay visitor.

PROPHYLAXIS

There are two strategies that I don't recommend for preventing travelers' diarrhea: antibiotics and antacids:

Prophylactic means "to prevent." For this strategy, you take something for the entire time you're abroad to prevent diarrhea. There are two ways to approach this: Either you take an antibiotic or Pepto-Bismol (bismuth subsalicylate [BSS]) tablets every day you're abroad. I recommend neither.

Antibiotics have side effects. It's true that if you take an appropriate antibiotic for your entire stay in a low-income nation, your risk of diarrhea lessens, but you may then suffer a side effect of the antibiotic: rash, stomach upset, or even diarrhea—the very thing you're trying to prevent. Also, antibiotics can cause vaginal yeast infections in women and can interact with most drugs. Given all the pros and all the cons, taking an antibiotic preventatively for an illness that is usually mild and self-limited is a poor option.

I have different reasons for advising you to stay away from prophylactic Pepto-Bismol. First off, does it work? The answer is yes. If you are sufficiently organized to ingest two caplets or chewable tablets or 30 ml of the liquid (2 tablespoons, or 6 teaspoons) four times a day, for your whole trip, your risk, as shown in multiple studies, will come down by about half—hardly a trivial reduction. However, few of us have the wherewithal to remember to take a drug four times a day for any prolonged period. Plus, there are side effects: Your tongue turns black (I'm serious), and your stool turns dark; it can also cause constipation and ringing in the ears. (These quickly resolve when you stop the Pepto-Bismol.) I suppose that if you do not mind chewing tablets four times a day for your trip, a black tongue, and weird poop, sure, take the Pepto-Bismol. But in my experience almost no one does this.

Pepto-Bismol should not be taken by pregnant women, people allergic to aspirin, children under age 12, those with chronic renal insufficiency, those taking another salicylate medicine (e.g., aspirin), and those taking certain other drugs (check with your physician or pharmacist).

Note: There are no data regarding taking bismuth subsalicylate for longer than four weeks.

For travelers at elevated risk for complications from travelers' diarrhea (e.g., those with inflammatory bowel disease or other chronic medical problems), an option is taking the antibiotic rifaximin (Xifaxan) preventively for the entire trip. This is a nonabsorbable antibiotic; it remains in your GI tract, and hence the rate of side effects is low. This is available by prescription only. *Note:* The use of rifaximin for prevention of travelers' diarrhea is not currently approved by the FDA. Also, currently, in the US its price is exorbitant.

CARRY-ALONG DRUGS FOR DIARRHEA

This is the option that I recommend: Carry a few antibiotic pills, and if you feel fine, take nothing.

In olden days (c. 1990), travel providers prescribed a sulfa-based drug, sulfamethoxazole/trimethoprim (Bactrim, Septra), which worked very nicely to hasten the return to normal bowel movements. However, bacteria quickly developed resistance to sulfa-based antibiotics. Then, for many years we used a drug in the fluoroquinolone category, such as ciprofloxacin (Cipro), but for reasons detailed below it has fallen out of favor. Now the most common antibiotic used for treatment of travelers' diarrhea is azithromycin.

TREATMENT OF TRAVELERS' DIARRHEA

MILD DIARRHEA (tolerable, not distressing, does not interfere with planned activities)

Taking an antibiotic is not advised.

Increase fluids by mouth.

Consider loperamide or Pepto-Bismol.

The loperamide dose is two tablets (4 mg) initially, then one tablet after each loose bowel movement, not to exceed eight tablets per twenty-four hours. *Note:* Loperamide should be avoided in children under age 6.

The Pepto-Bismol dose is two tablets up to four times a day until symptoms are resolving.

MODERATE DIARRHEA (distressing, or interferes with planned activities)

Increase fluids by mouth.

Consider antibiotic. The antibiotic of choice is usually azithromycin (500 mg per day for one to three days. The alternate dose of 1000 mg [one gram] causes a higher rate of GI upset). Other antibiotic options include ciprofloxacin (Cipro) and rifaximin (Xifaxan). *Note:* The fluoroquinolones, e. g. Cipro, are less effective than azithromycin in Southeast and South Asia.

Consider loperamide alone, without antibiotic. The initial dose is 4 mg, then 2 mg after each loose stool, not to exceed 16 mg in twenty-four hours.

SEVERE DIARRHEA (incapacitating, or completely prevents planned activities)

Increase fluids by mouth.

Take an antibiotic, usually azithromycin, 500 mg once per day for one to three days.

Consider loperamide in addition to the azithromycin.

DYSENTERY (blood in stool, often associated with fever)

Increase fluids by mouth.

For an antibiotic, azithromycin is the drug of choice. Either 1 gram once, or 500 mg once per day for three days.

Avoid loperamide.

Consider seeking medical attention for severe symptoms or if not improving.

Another treatment option is the antibiotic rifaximin. The treatment dose is 200 mg three times per day for three days.

In 2016 the FDA issued a warning regarding the side effects of fluoroquinolones, a category of antibiotics that includes ciprofloxacin (Cipro) and levofloxacin (Levaquin). The FDA warning stated that fluoroquinolones "are associated with disabling and potentially permanent serious side effects that can occur together. These side effects can involve the tendons, muscles, joints, nerves, and central nervous system." The risk of tendon injury (tendonitis or tendon rupture) is higher in those over age 60 and those taking steroids, such as prednisone, chronically.

Another reason to avoid taking fluoroquinolones is that these antibiotics have a greater effect on the body's natural GI microbiome (live organisms in the GI tract, many of which are beneficial) than do other antibiotics, such as azithromycin.

The FDA warning advised that for certain infections, including acute sinusitis, acute bronchitis, and uncomplicated urinary tract infections, an antibiotic other than a fluoroquinolone should be used if possible. The FDA warning did not address treatment of travelers' diarrhea, but travel medicine experts are in general agreement that drugs in this category should be avoided when possible. Cipro and other fluoroquinolones are still on the market, but their popularity is waning.

There are a few caveats that you must follow if you're going to use the carry-along strategy:

- Unlike other situations in which you use antibiotics, you stop taking the carry-along antibiotics as soon as you're better. For example, when you take azithromycin, usually a single 500 mg dose is sufficient, although you may take this once per day for up to three days.

- Only take the carry-along antibiotic and anti-motility drugs for "normal" diarrhea. If worrisome signs are present—such as significant abdominal pain—see a physician instead. If you're in some remote place, take the antibiotic on the way to seeing a doctor. Do not take loperamide if fever or blood in the stool is present.

- If you've taken antibiotics for two days and your diarrhea is not calming down, see a doctor. The vast majority of standard travelers' diarrhea due to ETEC will improve after a day or two; if you're not better, maybe something else is going on.

Backpackers and campers are at elevated risk for diarrhea caused by a protozoan organism, giardia. Antibiotics such as azithromycin do not work to cure this. Traditionally most doctors have prescribed metronidazole (Flagyl) for giardia; however, in recent years giardia has become increasingly resistant to this drug. For my patients with giardia, I usually prescribe tinidazole (Tindamax), 2 grams once. It has three advantages over metronidazole:

- There's less resistance to it.
- Its once-only dosing schedule is more convenient than that of metronidazole, which you have to take three times a day for several days.
- It has fewer side effects (e.g., less likelihood of stomach upset) than metronidazole.

But tinidazole also has its downside:

- It's more expensive than metronidazole.
- Potential side effects include itchiness, headache, and fatigue.
- As with metronidazole, you can't drink alcoholic beverages when you take tinidazole. If you do, you'll vomit for some time. (This is known as the "Antabuse-like" side effect.)

SAFE WATER

Several strategies can ensure that your drinking water is safe. All have pros and cons, all have their adherents and detractors. Bottled water, filters, boiling, adding iodine or chlorine, UV light—any is a reasonable choice. It may be optimal to use a combination of these options, depending on your circumstances.

Bottled Water

Bottled water is available in most places visited by tourists. If it's sealed when you buy it, the odds are good that it's safe to drink. Be suspicious of bottled water that is brought to your table already opened—it may or may not be safe. A drawback of this method is that it's less environmentally friendly than the following methods—you leave a trail of empty plastic bottles behind you.

Filters

Filters clear water of bacteria and larger organisms very nicely; they tend to be less helpful for viruses, which are much smaller. However, viruses are not a major cause of travelers' diarrhea, so this is a reasonable option. (If you use a reverse osmosis filter, it will remove viruses as well.) I do not like the weight and bulkiness of filters, so I do not use this strategy myself, but if this is your preference, go for it.

Boiling

Boiling kills all microorganisms that can give you diarrhea (with the exception of bacterial spores, which are not a common cause of diarrhea). And, despite what you may read, you do not need to boil your water for any specified amount of time—just bring it to a boil, then let it cool. However, in hotels or on the road, you often do not have the means to boil water, so you probably should not rely on this as your lone strategy.

Note: If you're packing an electric water pot, be sure to take both an electrical adapter (with prongs for foreign outlets) and a converter (for foreign electrical currents).

Although it is true that the boiling temperature of water decreases with increased altitude, the temperature of boiling water at altitude is still sufficiently high to kill microorganisms.

Iodine or Chlorine (Halogenation)

This is the method I utilize. Even if you're planning on utilizing one of the other strategies, consider taking a bottle of iodine pills as a backup method. Advantages of this method are that iodine tablets are inexpensive and lightweight.

Iodine kills bacteria and viruses. Some encapsulated organisms (e.g., Cryptosporidium) can survive iodine, but they are not common causes of travelers' diarrhea.

Add a single iodine tablet to a liter or quart of water and wait twenty minutes. Some people do not like the taste of iodine-treated water, but I don't mind it. If the taste of iodine bothers you, adding a smidge of vitamin C (50 mg/liter of water) after the required contact time removes the iodine taste. Remember to pack a clean bottle for this purpose.

A Final Caveat

One more caveat regarding travelers' diarrhea (one that many physicians and other health personnel are unaware of): Anything that reduces the acidity of your stomach will increase your susceptibility to travelers' diarrhea. Stomach acid is a major barrier against microbes; the extreme acidity of your stomach kills almost all of them. Thus, if you routinely take an antacid, such as Maalox or Mylanta, or a medication that reduces stomach acid, such as cimetidine (Tagamet), ranitidine (Zantac), famotidine (Pepcid), or omeprazole (Prilosec), your odds of getting the trots while abroad are increased.

Food Safety Q&A

Q **What if a restaurant advertises that all its foods are cleaned in sterile water? Is it safe to eat there?**
A Maybe.

Q **What about organic food. Any safer?**
A Maybe. I would avoid unpasteurized milk, which can spread brucellosis, tuberculosis, the life-threatening strain of E. coli, and other serious illnesses. Also avoid unpasteurized juice, which can transmit any number of troublemakers, including Salmonella.

Q **Since anything that reduces stomach acidity will increase my odds of travelers' diarrhea, should I stop my antacid or other acid-reducing drug prior to my trip?**

A In most cases, no. Especially if you have untoward symptoms that are controlled by your medication, I think you should continue it. There is no point in going on vacation and having every meal give you heartburn.

Q So then should I avoid low-income nations?

A It's your call, but I would say no. Still, I would certainly travel with one of the prescription drugs that shortens the duration of travelers' diarrhea, as already noted.

Q Are there potential downsides to taking carry-along antibiotics?

A You bet. In fact, if any physician ever tells you that any drug treatment never has any side effects for anyone, get a new doctor.

Any antibiotic can cause a rash, stomach upset, or diarrhea in and of itself, as well as a host of other side effects. Most people do not get these, but a significant minority do. Overall, most people who take an appropriate antibiotic for travelers' diarrhea feel better sooner than those who do not.

Q Is every case of diarrhea abroad due to travelers' diarrhea?

A No. Travelers' diarrhea is defined as diarrhea caused by an ingested microorganism—usually a bacterium—that affects the lining of the gut. Many other processes can lead to diarrhea, including pyelonephritis (kidney infection), appendicitis, and malaria. If symptoms are present that are outside the realm of ordinary and uncomplicated travelers' diarrhea (e.g., fever, blood in stool, significant abdominal pain, diarrhea that doesn't resolve after two days of antibiotics), see a physician.

Q What if I have something really serious—such as appendicitis or malaria—and I mistakenly think it's travelers' diarrhea? Couldn't I be delaying needed treatment by taking carry-along antibiotics?

A In theory, yes. In practice, however, people seem to know when they have uncomplicated travelers' diarrhea and when something more dire is going on. Travelers should have a low threshold for seeking medical care should their symptoms seem more alarming than garden-variety *turista*. But as I say, travelers seem fairly savvy on this point.

Q Perhaps I should bring more than one drug—azithromycin for bacterial causes, as well as something for giardia?

A This would work well if you pack a microscope, culture media, and a trained lab tech, but it won't if you don't. You cannot tell what the cause of your diarrhea is from symptoms. It is true, for example, that giardia causes particularly foul-smelling farts and belching that smells like sulfur—but this is not specific for giardia. Similarly, Campylobacter causes symptoms that are in general more severe than those caused by ETEC, but you cannot reliably tell which bug is tormenting you by the symptoms. I advise you to take a single drug—usually azithromycin—and if that first drug doesn't work, see a physician.

Q Do I need to carry special salts to make up an oral rehydration therapy (ORT) to drink as a fluid replacement in case I get travelers' diarrhea?

A For most people, no. Travelers' diarrhea is not a dehydrating diarrhea; people with travelers' diarrhea do not tend to get dehydrated (unless it is accompanied by prolonged vomiting, which is uncommon), and simple fluid replacement—water, weak tea—will usually suffice. However, this is not true at the extremes of age. In the very young (under age 2) and the elderly, travelers' diarrhea can indeed be a dehydrating diarrhea. So very young and elderly international travelers should indeed carry an ORT solution.

The ORT can also be assembled on the spot. To one liter of clean water, add one level teaspoon of salt and eight level teaspoons of sugar. Adding half a cup of orange juice or half a mashed banana to each liter adds potassium and improves taste.

Q While I'm recovering from travelers' diarrhea, should I rest my gut? Is a liquids-only diet best?

A In olden days (say, thirty years ago) physicians thought that an injured gut healed best with a bland diet: liquids, toast, not much else. More recent research shows that healing guts do very well with a variety of foods and do not need to be rested. Rapidly resuming a full diet may actually hasten resolution of symptoms.

Q What about probiotics?

A Taking probiotic supplements preventatively has not been shown to reduce risk of travelers' diarrhea. However, doing so has been shown to reduce the risk of antibiotic-associated diarrhea. Thus, if you're taking an antibiotic for any reason, taking a probiotic (e.g., *Lactobacillus* GG) concurrently will reduce the risk of diarrhea as a side effect of the antibiotic. Don't take probiotics if you are pregnant or immunocompromised, or have a prosthetic heart valve, inflammatory bowel disease (Crohn's disease or ulcerative colitis), or an ostomy.

Q Isn't there anything I can do that will guarantee I will not get diarrhea?

A No. Diarrhea is a common travel malady in low-income nations, and your control is finite.

Q I don't want to take an antibiotic.

A Yours is a reasonable attitude. Most travelers' diarrhea resolves in a few days without treatment. Usually, taking an antibiotic is an option, not a necessity.

Travelers' Diarrhea Myths

"If I'm careful in my choice of food and beverages, I will not get this."
This is partially true. You can—possibly, slightly—reduce your risk of travelers' diarrhea by choosing food that's boiled or cooked in some other way, but even cautious eaters develop diarrhea. Most studies have found a minimal to negligible benefit from eating cautiously.

"It's normal to get travelers' diarrhea. When people from poor countries come to the high-income nations, they get diarrhea too."
It's not so. The average kid in the slums of Lima, Peru, develops diarrhea about seven times per year; this is far higher than the rate of diarrhea in children in more affluent nations. Visitors to the US get diarrhea at about the same rate as do residents of the US—that is, not often.

"If I eat enough garlic or if I put enough lemon juice on my food, I never get sick."
It's hard to argue with success, but no study has shown that these measures are protective.

"I always know exactly what food or drink made me sick."
You can't know the culprit with certainty. It's human nature to speculate, but this is guesswork. The incubation period for travelers' diarrhea can be as little as a few hours, or as long as several weeks.

Travelers' Diarrhea: Incubation Periods

Food poisoning (bacterial toxin)	a few hours
Bacterial and viral pathogens	6–72 hours
Protozoan pathogens (e.g., giardia)	1–2 weeks

Hence when you get travelers' diarrhea, everything you've consumed for the previous several weeks is suspect.

For those with a fascination with poop and its aberrations, I refer you to Ericsson, DuPont, and Steffen's 293-page, well-formed *Travelers' Diarrhea,* 2nd edition (Hamilton, ON: B.C. Decker Inc., 2008).

Gut Microbiome Q&A

Q **What is the gut microbiome?**

A The gut microbiome refers to the large, complex mix of live bacteria and other microorganisms that reside in our GI tracts. Healthy adults harbor more than one thousand different species of bacteria.

Q **What is the role of the gut microbiome?**

A These microorganisms contribute to metabolic function, protect against pathogens, and educate the immune system—in fact they affect, directly or indirectly, most of our physiologic functions. Gut microbiota play a significant role in host digestion and nutrition and can generate nutrients from foodstuffs otherwise indigestible by the host.

Q **What determines the constituent organisms within a person's gut microbiome?**

A This is multifactorial. Not only diet but also gender and level of education attained affect the organisms. Family members are likely to share species.

Q **What is dysbiosis?**

A Dysbiosis refers to a microbiota community that is associated with a particular disease state. However, it is difficult to determine whether the patterns noted with particular diseases are a cause or a result of the illness. Obesity, diabetes, rheumatoid arthritis, and colorectal cancer are a few of the medical conditions that are associated with particular patterns of gut organisms. Ongoing research is exploring the potential link between gut microbiota and cardiovascular disease.

Q What is the effect of antibiotics on the gut microbiome?

A Taking an antibiotic is associated with reduced microbiota diversity—that is, a lessened number of types of organisms.

Q Can the gut microbiome be related to mood and mood disorders?

A Recent studies have shown that organisms in the gut microbiome can activate neural pathways and central nervous system (CNS) signaling systems. The gut–brain axis appears to be bidirectional: gut microorganisms create neuroactive chemicals, including neurotransmitters, that act on the brain; and the brain influences GI and immune functions that control the gut's mix of microorganisms. It is interesting to note that probiotics have been shown to reduce anxiety and stress in mice.

Q What is the effect of travel on the gut microbiome?

A Travel alters gut bacteria. A study of Finnish travelers, primarily in tropical and subtropical regions, found that during travel 21% were colonized with the multiple-drug resistant (MDR) intestinal bacteria Extended-Spectrum Beta-Lactamase-Producing *Enterobacteriaceae* (ESBL-PE). (Pre-travel, only about 1% of travelers tested positive for this.)

The following factors have been associated with returning with this MDR bacterium:

- Travel to low-income nations (particularly South Asia; no cases were identified among visitors to Europe, Australia, or the Americas)
- Having travelers' diarrhea
- Taking an antibiotic for travelers' diarrhea

The highest risk of acquiring this bacterium was seen in those taking both an antibiotic and loperamide for travelers' diarrhea. Taking loperamide alone did not elevate risk.

Note: Taking an antimalarial was *not* found to be a risk factor.

These bacteria are not usually associated with symptoms in healthy adults, and their presence in the GI tract is transient. Their impact on health is unknown.

Diseases for Which
There Are No Vaccines

The Bottom Line

Humans are at risk for, by one count, 1,415 infectious diseases; vaccines exist for only a handful. The strategies outlined below can reduce your chances of acquiring many of the diseases for which there are no vaccines.

Dengue Fever

Dengue fever (pronounced DEN-gee fever; the "g" is hard) is caused by a virus that is transmitted by mosquitoes; it is present throughout the tropics. Its name derives from the Swahili *ki denga pepo*, variously translated as "it is a sudden overtaking by a spirit" and "cramplike seizure caused by an evil spirit." Treatment is supportive (rest, hydration, painkillers)—physicians try to make you comfortable until the infection resolves.

Dengue is a crummy illness; the fact that it's known as break-bone fever should give you some idea. You ache—you ache like you've never ached before. Often the headache is centered directly behind your eyes, as though someone were boring a subway tunnel through your head. People say it feels as though knitting needles have been driven into every joint in their bodies. This goes on for some days. You have high fevers; you may get a rash.

Since there is no vaccine available to most travelers, is this a random disease—some folks get it and most do not and you have no control? No! You have *huge* control over this. You can bring your risk down to almost zero. Think: vector = mosquitoes. If mosquitoes do not bite you, you will not get this.

So, how do you avoid getting bitten by mosquitoes, given that they are present practically everywhere in the tropics? Simple: Follow the same bug-avoidance measures as for malaria (see chapter 3):

- Apply DEET (20%–50%) or picaridin (20%) to exposed skin.
- Apply permethrin to all clothes.
- Sleep under a bed net, preferably one treated with permethrin.
- Wear long sleeves and pants.

Any one of the preceding measures offers some protection; the combo of all four makes you nearly a no-bug zone.

The mosquitoes that transmit dengue (and chikungunya and the Zika virus) bite during daylight hours (and dawn and dusk); using these measures during these hours is particularly important for the prevention of these three diseases. However, the mosquitoes that transmit malaria bite at night (and dawn and dusk), so there's really no time during which you can be blasé about personal protection measures.

Travelers who suspect that they have dengue fever should avoid taking aspirin or other nonsteroidal anti-inflammatory medications (e.g., ibuprofen [Advil, Motrin], naproxen [Aleve]) as these may worsen dengue's tendency to interfere with blood's ability to clot. It's fine to take acetaminophen (Tylenol) for dengue.

Actually, there is a vaccine for dengue fever, Dengvaxia, first licensed for use in Mexico in 2015 for people ages 9 to 45; it has also been approved in the Philippines, Indonesia, Brazil, El Salvador, Costa Rica, and Paraguay. It is not currently available in the US or other high-income nations. Given that the vaccine series consists of three doses over twelve months, it is not practical for most travelers to receive this vaccine.

Recent research has shown that this vaccine is safer for people who have already had dengue fever. Specifically, those who have never had dengue fever who receive this vaccine and then contract dengue fever are at higher risk for severe illness and hospitalization relative to those who have had dengue fever, then receive the vaccine, then contract dengue fever. Hence, only those with laboratory-confirmed prior infection with dengue should get this vaccine.

DENGUE HEMORRHAGIC FEVER

The cause of dengue hemorrhagic fever remains controversial and speculative. Of the five similar but distinct serotypes of dengue fever, four were known for many years, and a fifth was discovered in 2013. If you develop dengue fever, you will subsequently be immune for life to the specific serotype that caused your infection. However, if you then develop an infection with one of the other four serotypes, not only are you not immune, but you are at increased risk for dengue hemorrhagic fever. This mechanism is known as antibody-dependent enhancement. However, this is only one of the many causal factors that have been identified. Some strains of dengue can cause dengue hemorrhagic syndrome in primary infections. Some genetic factors seem to predispose. In Southeast Asia, children are at higher risk to develop dengue hemorrhagic fever, whereas in the Americas all ages are at risk.

Dengue Fever Q&A

Q Given increasing urbanization, is dengue fever on the decline?

A To the contrary, it is an emerging disease—that is, it's increasingly common. Rates of dengue increased thirtyfold between

1960 and 2010. The World Health Organization (WHO) estimates that fifty million to a hundred million cases occur around the world each year, causing half a million cases of dengue hemorrhagic fever (see the following) and twenty-two thousand deaths.

Q Is death from dengue fever likely?

A Usually, no. Usually you're miserable and you have the worst headache of your life, but you do not die. However, there is also a severe form of dengue, called dengue hemorrhagic fever. The mechanism that causes dengue hemorrhagic fever is controversial (see sidebar). In dengue hemorrhagic fever, in addition to the usual misery of dengue, your blood doesn't clot normally and you may spontaneously bleed from your nose, rectum, and elsewhere. About 5% of people who develop dengue hemorrhagic fever die from it. Treatment is again supportive—we try to keep you comfortable while your body battles the infection.

Q I think I had dengue fever. Should I be tested to see which of the five types I had, so that I can avoid getting a second, different type, and thus avoid risk of dengue hemorrhagic syndrome?

A Good question. The bottom line is that most tropical medicine specialists do not recommend routine serologic testing in people who have had, or people who may have had, dengue fever. The epidemiology of dengue is complex. Outbreaks are often of more than one serotype, and different geographic locations have epidemics of different serotypes from year to year. The reason that this question has a complex or equivocal answer is that, in theory, indeed you could find out which of the five serotypes you were infected with, then avoid travel to areas with epidemics of the other types. However, given the shifting nature of dengue epidemics, this is close to impossible. Probably the best strategy is to be near fanatical about anti-mosquito personal protection measures (PPMs) (see chapter 3), and, should you contract dengue regardless, continue to be maniacal regarding PPMs.

Leptospirosis

Leptospirosis is the most common zoonosis (disease spread from animals to people). Caused by a bacterium that is passed in the urine of animals, most commonly rodents, leptospirosis is acquired by exposure of contaminated water to mouth, eyes, nose, and breaks in the skin; it can also be acquired via inhalation of an aerosol as might occur in an abattoir. Swimming in contaminated fresh water is the most common mode of transmission to travelers. Leptospirosis is present throughout the tropics and subtropics; it is present in the Hawaiian Islands, particularly the two islands with the highest rainfall: Hawaii (the Big Island) and Kauai. In people who live in endemic areas, it is an occupational illness, seen in rice and sugarcane workers, sewage workers, and miners. This illness is probably underdiagnosed, as many doctors do not consider it when they see a patient with fever and jaundice.

After an incubation period that usually lasts between one and two weeks, but may be as brief as two days or as long as one month, the illness starts with the sudden onset of high fever, chills, and headache; many people progress to jaundice. Over 90% of cases are not too terrible and resolve without treatment. But in a minority of people symptoms are severe, often with jaundice; these cases can be life threatening. The illness may be biphasic—that is, with two periods of symptoms separated by a period during which the person feels fine. These people have a fever and feel achy for three to seven days, then feel fine for up to a month, then develop severe symptoms, including jaundice.

Once the diagnosis is made, treatment with common and inexpensive antibiotics (e.g., penicillin, amoxicillin, doxycycline), if begun sufficiently early, reduces the duration and severity of illness.

Leptospirosis Q&A

Q **I'm going into the ocean but not into fresh water. Do I have to worry about leptospirosis?**

A No. The bacteria that causes it cannot live in salt water.

Q **I'm going to an area that has chloroquine-sensitive malaria, so I'm taking chloroquine or Plaquenil for malaria prevention. I'll also be rafting in rivers. What should I do?**

A Switch your antimalarial to doxycycline. This will prevent malaria and prevent leptospirosis as well.

LEPTOSPIROSIS IN BORNEO: ECO-CHALLENGE SABAH 2000

In 2000, 304 athletes from twenty-six countries, including competitors from twenty-nine US states, converged on northern Malaysian Borneo to compete in Eco-Challenge Sabah 2000, a ten-day multisport endurance event. The contestants trekked through jungle, mountain biked, spelunked, and swam and kayaked in both fresh and salt water. After the event they returned to their respective twenty-six countries. A few days later, one by one, many started to develop high fevers, nausea, and headaches; several developed jaundice.

The GeoSentinel network, an international surveillance network of travel clinics, quickly recognized an uptick in leptospirosis cases and notified the CDC in the US. The CDC found that 42% of the athletes they contacted had leptospirosis, 36% of whom required hospitalization. Those taking doxycycline for malaria prevention were protected from leptospirosis.

Other outbreaks of leptospirosis have occurred in athletes. In 1998, more than 110 triathletes who swam in lakes in Illinois and Wisconsin in two separate events developed leptospirosis. As is often the case, these outbreaks followed heavy rains. (Imagine all that animal urine being carried to the lake by rainwater.)

If you are going to be engaged in a freshwater sport in the tropics, such as swimming or river rafting, you may want to consider taking an antibiotic such as doxycycline prophylactically (preventatively). The dose of doxycycline for leptospirosis prevention is different from that for malaria prevention. For leptospirosis prevention, you take 200 mg once per week; for malaria prevention you take 100 mg once per day. The malaria regimen is sufficient to prevent leptospirosis, but the leptospirosis regimen is not sufficient to prevent malaria, so if you are attempting to prevent both, utilize the malaria regimen of 100 mg once per day.

Hepatitis C

Hepatitis C is spread by blood: You can contract it from a reused needle or a blood transfusion. Unlike hepatitis B, it is only very rarely spread by sex. Infection is usually lifelong, and in 20% to 30% of cases progresses to cirrhosis. Until recently, hepatitis C was the most common reason in the US that people needed liver transplants (current most common cause: non-alcoholic steatohepatitis [NASH] cirrhosis).

Avoidance: Avoid needle pokes, tattoos, piercings, and blood transfusions in low- and middle-income nations.

HIV

The drugs for HIV are better than they used to be, but there is still no vaccine and no cure. Multiple studies have shown that the risk of acquiring HIV on holiday is markedly higher than the odds of contracting it at home; this is probably related to "holiday behavior," by which I mean people who vacation not infrequently and have new sexual partners.

Condoms: If you think there is even a teeny chance of you having a new partner while abroad, take some condoms with you. These should be latex and manufactured in a high-income nation. There are no restrictions on carrying condoms through Customs.

In many low-income nations, hospitals and medical clinics reuse needles. Often the needle is cleaned between patients, but this may not fully sterilize the needle. That needle then has the potential to transmit a number of incurable illnesses, including, but not limited to, hepatitis B, hepatitis C, and HIV/AIDS.

I admit that I am probably being unfairly and overly inclusive. Many clinics and hospitals in low- and middle-income nations, particularly in urban centers, use a new needle for each patient. But given that the stakes are so high, I'd err on the conservative side. This should be your strategy outside high-income nations: If a doctor or nurse or anyone else tells you that you need a shot, blood draw, transfusion, or fluid by IV, say thanks but no thanks—unless you are in truly dire straits.

Generally, it's no big deal to avoid shots. Most antibiotics can be given by mouth; most diarrhea can be treated with fluids by mouth. There is in many cultures something of a "cult of the injection"—many providers will fear that you may feel that you haven't had truly good care if they do not give you a shot. If you have sufficient wits about you to be concerned about the injection, you probably aren't sick enough to need it. Admittedly, the needle may very well be sterile, and you may offend providers by intimating that their needles might be contaminated, but better that than dealing with a lifetime of illness.

Similarly, I strongly advise that travelers avoid all other services and procedures that entail something sharp. You want your face, legs, or elsewhere shaved? Fine—buy a plastic blister-packed razor at a supermarket or drug store and do it yourself. You want a new piercing or tattoo? Get it done in a high-income nation prior to or after your trip. Bottom line: Reused needles can transmit lethal illnesses. Avoid all needles, even ones that are purportedly sterile, outside of industrialized nations.

STDs Other Than HIV

With the exceptions of hepatitis B and human papilloma virus (HPV), there are no vaccines for sexually transmitted diseases (STDs). See the section on sexual activity in chapter 12.

Avoidance: This is the same as previously listed for HIV.

Lyme Disease

The vaccine for Lyme disease was taken off the market in 2002. This illness, spread by ticks, is more common in temperate regions (e.g., the US, Scotland, and southern Sweden). Symptoms include rash, arthritis, and heart and nervous system disease.

Avoidance: Avoid tick bites. While hiking, tuck your pants' cuffs into your boots, wear a DEET repellent, and after hiking perform a whole-body examination for ticks with the help of a full-length mirror or a close friend.

Zika Virus

Prior to 2015, outbreaks of Zika virus occurred in several countries in Africa, Southeast Asia, and some Pacific islands. In May 2015, it was detected in Brazil; it quickly spread to essentially all countries in Central America, South America, and the Caribbean. Activity peaked in 2016, with markedly fewer cases in 2017.

Only about 20% of people who become infected with the Zika virus have symptoms; in 80%, infection is asymptomatic (and can be detected only by specific laboratory testing). Those with symptoms develop fever, rash, joint pain, and conjunctivitis (pink eye). These symptoms are similar to those seen in dengue fever and chikungunya. Additionally, infection with the Zika virus in pregnant women markedly elevates the risk of microcephaly, a condition in which newborns have small heads and underdeveloped brains.

Zika is primarily transmitted by mosquitoes, but it also can be spread by sex, from a pregnant woman to her fetus, and by blood transfusion.

Avoidance: Travelers can markedly reduce the risk of Zika virus infection when traveling in endemic areas by the use of the usual anti-mosquito measures: applying DEET or picaridin to exposed skin, applying permethrin to clothing, and sleeping under bed nets. Use of these measures reduces risk of dengue fever by as much as 99%; the protection is probably similar for Zika virus.

When possible, pregnant women, or potentially pregnant women, should avoid travel to Zika-endemic regions. Furthermore, men with pregnant or potentially pregnant partners should also avoid travel to Zika-endemic regions.

If a couple is attempting to conceive, they should wait at least eight weeks after the woman's last potential exposure (or after onset of symptoms if any) before attempting conception; they should wait at least three months after the man's last potential exposure (or onset of symptoms if any). During this waiting period, either abstinence or condoms should be employed.

Chikungunya

Like dengue fever, chikungunya is a viral illness transmitted by mosquitoes. Symptoms include fever, joint pain, headache, muscle pain, swelling of the joints, and rash. Most patients fully recover, but joint pain can last months or even years.

As with dengue fever, chikungunya's geographic range is expanding. Outbreaks have occurred in countries in Africa, Asia, Europe, and the Indian and Pacific Oceans. In 2013 chikungunya was detected in several islands in the Caribbean.

Risk reduction is the same as for dengue and Zika.

Bird Flu

Avian flu, or bird flu, is caused by viruses that ordinarily only infect birds. However, since 1997 avian influenza viruses have infected a small number of people. Among the avian influenza viruses that have infected people since 1997, H5N1 has been the most common. One reason that the number of those affected remains relatively low is that sustained human-to-human transmission of the virus has not occurred. The odds of avian influenza viruses mutating such that person-to-person transmission occurs are unknown.

Bird Flu Q&A

Q What countries have had human cases of avian flu?
A Since 2003, there have been more than eight hundred cases of bird flu in people. The fatality rate has been 53%. Cases have been reported from more than sixty countries, but most cases have been detected in fifteen countries in Asia, Africa, the Pacific, Europe, and the Middle East.

Q I'm thinking of visiting a country with ongoing avian influenza transmission. Should I go?
A The CDC does not currently recommend that travelers avoid any country because of avian influenza. They do advise that travelers avoid handling live or dead birds or surfaces that might be contaminated with bird secretions or feces. Additionally, travelers should avoid poultry farms and bird markets in countries with ongoing transmission.

Q What is the risk of bird flu to the international traveler?
A It appears to be minuscule. The majority of people who contract bird flu are those who have close and ongoing contact with birds, such as chicken farmers and duck vendors.

Q What are the symptoms of bird flu infection in humans?

A Symptoms range from typical influenza symptoms—fever, muscle aches, cough—to severe respiratory illness and other life-threatening complications.

Q Can I be immunized for bird flu?

A As of 2018, there are no vaccines on the market. It is thought that a vaccine will probably not be available early in a pandemic, should one occur.

Q Are poultry and eggs safe to eat in countries with ongoing avian influenza transmission?

A Yes, if well cooked.

Q Are there any measures that might reduce my risk of this illness?

A Frequent hand washing with soap and water, or an alcohol-based hand sanitizer gel, probably reduces risk.

Q Should I take an antiviral medication such as Tamiflu (oseltamivir) with me when I travel to a country with ongoing bird flu transmission?

A The benefit of Tamiflu for bird flu is unknown. Some travel medicine providers feel that it's reasonable to carry a course of Tamiflu when you travel in countries endemic for bird flu. My thought is that it's difficult for the traveler to discern if fever and aches are due to influenza or something else, so I don't routinely advise carrying it.

Q Just how worried should I be about bird flu?

A Influenza pandemics—worse than usual flu seasons—tend to occur three or four times per century. During the twentieth century, three pandemics occurred: in 1918–1919, 1957–1958, and

1968–1969. There will certainly be more in the future. Of note, the most severe pandemic, which occurred in 1918–1919, was caused by an avian influenza virus that mutated such that it was easily transmitted between people. The timing of the next epidemic and whether its cause will be a traditional human influenza virus or an avian influenza virus are unknown.

Really Rare, Really Bad

The Bottom Line

All of the causes of illness and injury described in this chapter are extremely rare in tourists and other short-stay visitors to middle- and low-income nations.

THE NEXT TIME you read about travelers being killed by volcanic ash, or devoured by a lion, recall that only one in one hundred thousand international travelers dies while abroad. Nonetheless, I will discuss a few rare conditions and scenarios that you want to experience via your reading only.

Cholera

Outbreaks of cholera, a diarrheal disease spread by food and water, occur regularly around the world. Cholera has the potential to cause death from dehydration. An ongoing epidemic in Haiti that began in 2010 has killed more than seven thousand people and sickened hundreds of thousands. Cholera is extremely rare in visitors from high-income nations.

Avoidance: Do not drink river water. It's sad to say, but every river contains the sewage of someone upstream. Avoid food and beverages from street stands. Follow dietary guidelines discussed in chapter 4.

A cholera vaccine was approved by the FDA in 2016; it is indicated for those at elevated risk, such as healthcare workers in cholera-endemic regions (see chapter 2).

Chagas Disease (American Trypanosomiasis)

Chagas disease is not rare among residents of Latin America; it is estimated that six million to eight million people are infected in twenty-one countries in Central America and South America, causing about eighteen thousand deaths per year. Spread by the bite of a bloodsucking insect vector—Trypanosoma cruzi, one of the reduviid bugs—Chagas disease causes chronic changes to the heart and GI tract; sudden death from ventricular fibrillation is the most common cause of death.

Avoidance: This illness is phenomenally rare in tourists. Reduviid bugs live in the recesses of roofs and walls of mud huts. Don't sleep in mud huts; if you do, sleep under a mosquito net.

Kuru

Kuru is a fatal, progressive, neurological disease formerly seen in the Fore (pronounced FOUR-ay) people of the highlands of New Guinea. *Kuru* means "trembling with fear" in the Fore language. Those stricken with kuru suffered headache and joint pains followed by difficulty walking. This progressed to a tremor so severe that sitting upright was impossible. It invariably led to death within six to twenty-four months.

Epidemiological research showed the disease to be due to a small infectious particle, a prion, that infected the brain. The disease was spread by the ritual eating of departed relatives' brains. The disease was halted when the Fore followed epidemiologists' advice to stop this practice.

Avoidance: Do not eat anyone's brain, even if you knew them well. Remember, when you eat someone's brain, you're eating not only their brain but the brain of everyone they've eaten.

Rat Lungworm

The host of this parasite is the rat; snails and slugs transmit the illness to people who either ingest snails or slugs or consume produce contaminated by same. Symptoms include headache, fever, stiff neck, and meningitis (inflammation of the lining of the brain), which can be life threatening. Sometimes GI symptoms occur, including abdominal pain, nausea, and vomiting.

This parasite is most commonly transmitted in Southeast Asia and tropical Pacific islands; it also occurs in the Caribbean, Australia, and some regions of Africa. Currently in Hawaii 80% of land snails carry this parasite. The geographic range of the parasite appears to be expanding.

Avoidance: In endemic areas, avoid raw or undercooked slugs and snails; wash and/or heat (to at least 165°F [74°C]) fresh produce prior to consumption.

Volcanoes

If you're struck by a big blurp of lava, well, let's just say you won't be going through the Kübler-Ross stages of grief. In a 1999 article, researchers in Japan described the deaths of six climbers on Mount Aso, an active volcano in the Kumamoto prefecture, Japan. All six were within 800 feet (250 meters) of the crater lip when they met their end. Death was not due to lava but to inhalation of volcanic gases. In 2014, sixty-three hikers were killed when Mount Ontake (the second-highest volcano in Japan, after Mount Fuji) erupted.

Avoidance: Generally speaking, active volcanoes aren't subtle and are easily avoided by travelers who want to live into their senior years.

Nonetheless, a small number of volcano nuts enjoy getting right to the lip of active volcanoes. Enjoy volcanoes from a distance.

Being Eaten by a Lion

A 1999 article in the *Journal of Travel Medicine* described the deaths of four tourists in South Africa who were killed by lions. Significantly, three of the four were killed as they approached the lions on foot, as if to pet them. Now, folks, when you look at lions you may see placid animals in repose, but when they see you, they see a hamburger. You will not have time to explain your affinity for threatened species or hum "Born Free" before you become a snack.

SOSSUSVLEI

Some years back I went on a three-day guided camping tour of Sossusvlei, a clay pan in Namibia's central Namib Desert. I wanted to see the massive sand dunes, said by some to be the tallest in the world. The dunes, situated in the Namib-Naukluft National Park, are vast and red; some reach 900 feet (275 meters) in height.

On the first evening, I laid my sleeping bag on the sand. Our young Namibian tour guide, Ivan, said, "No, better to sleep in a tent or on top of the van."

"Why?"

"Could be creepy-crawlies."

I slept on the roof of the Land Cruiser. My evening was uneventful. When I returned, I entered *Sossusvlei* and *camping safety* into a search engine and found reports of hyenas biting overnight campers on their faces as they slept on the open ground. I bring this up not to say that camping in Africa is intrinsically dangerous but to suggest that when your guide gives advice, it is usually prudent to follow it.

Avoidance: At the game parks, do what the drivers do. Do they get out of the vans while in sight of lions? Or hippos or elephants or Cape buffaloes? No. Also, a small number of lion attacks have occurred when lions pounced through open car windows. Windows of vehicles in game parks should remain closed.

Travelers

Women

The Bottom Line

- Many infections, including influenza, malaria, and dengue fever, are more severe in pregnant women; hence appropriate immunization, use of an antimalarial, and personal protection measures (bug repellent, etc.) are particularly important during pregnancy.
- If you're prone to bladder or yeast infections, you can ask your pre-travel provider or usual physician for prescriptions for medications for as-needed use.
- If you are of childbearing years, not using birth control, and might have sex with a new partner, bring birth control. Also consider bringing a form of emergency (post–unprotected sex) contraception.

OF THOSE TAKING cultural, adventure, or nature trips, 75% are women. In fact, the average adventure traveler is a forty-seven-year-old woman.

Security

An unfortunate reality of international travel is that women, particularly when traveling alone, are more at risk for violation of their personal safety than are men. A 2013 study of 6,502 British and German travelers to Mediterranean resorts found that sexual harassment was more likely in travelers who were female, younger, frequently drunk on holiday, cocaine users, and attracted to bars where people get drunk.

Listen to your gut, by which I mean that if your general vibe is that the situation is dodgy—potentially unsafe, potentially unstable, potentially threatening—you should leave. In addition, take the following precautions:

Talk with hotel staff about local safety, including parts of town to avoid.

Do not wear expensive clothing or accessories.

Keep valuables (passport, credit cards) in a money belt. If you do carry a bag, use a cross-body bag that rests in front of you.

Carry a cell phone. Call your carrier prior to your trip to make sure coverage is available in your destinations (and to check on charges). Another option is to purchase a cell phone with an airtime card at your destination. This is relatively cheap in most low-income nations.

Avoid walking alone at night. Do not accept food or drink from strangers. Be particularly alert at nightclubs; do not leave your drink unattended, as some malefactor could spike it.

Do not accept rides from strangers, however helpful they might seem.

The US State Department website advises, "Be cautious when sharing information about your plans and itinerary with strangers. Don't feel the need to be overly polite if you are bothered by someone. Although it may seem rude to be unfriendly to a stranger, creating boundaries to protect yourself is important. Use facial expressions, body language, and a firm voice to fend off any unwanted attention."

First, some terminology:

burka: a long, loose garment covering the whole body from head to feet; the most concealing of Islamic veils; often with a mesh screen to see through

chador: a long, loose robe that covers the entire body and head; a full body cloak

hijab: a headscarf

kameez: a long shirt; commonly worn throughout the Indian subcontinent

niqab: a veil for the face; leaves the area around the eyes uncovered

shalwar kameez: baggy trousers

It is not necessary for women visitors to wear these specific items of clothing, but it is prudent and respectful in Muslim-majority countries, as in many other regions, to dress conservatively, covering arms and legs with loose clothing. Loose clothing has the additional advantage of being more comfortable in the heat. Also, covering one's hair with a scarf is said to help prevent unwanted attention from men. Covering hair with a scarf when visiting a mosque is a must.

Menstruation

Menstrual cycles during travel may become irregular or cease for reasons other than pregnancy. Changes in sleep pattern, an altered level of activity, increased stress, and illness can result in a cycle other than your baseline pattern. Your usual form of menstrual supplies may not be available overseas; pack accordingly.

Some women find it convenient to not have periods while traveling. Discuss options with your doctor prior to your trip. There is not a physiologic need for a period. For those taking the birth control pill, avoiding periods can be accomplished by skipping the inactive pills.

Many types of birth control pills contain twenty-one days of active pills followed by seven days of inactive pills. On day twenty-two of the cycle, instead of taking the first inactive pill, you take the first day of the next pack of twenty-one active pills. Breakthrough bleeding may occur, but this usually reduces over time.

Some birth control pills, known as extended cycle or continuous birth control pills, are specifically designed to lengthen the time between periods.

Seasonale, Jolessa, and Quasense are extended cycle pills: active pills are taken continuously for twelve weeks, followed by one week of inactive pills. Your period occurs during week thirteen, about once every three months. With Seasonique and Camrese, similarly, active pills are taken for twelve weeks. Then you would take low-dose estrogen pills for one week, during which the period occurs. The advantage of taking low-dose estrogen pills, as opposed to inactive pills, for week thirteen is that bleeding, bloating, and other side effects of the hormone-free interval are reduced.

Amethyst contains low doses of both progesterone and estrogen; it is designed to be taken continuously. There are no hormone-free intervals results—hence, no periods.

Contraception

A plethora of options are available for avoiding pregnancy, including birth control pills, intrauterine devices (IUDs), implants, and injections. All have pros and cons, all are markedly effective at preventing unwanted pregnancy.

Specific birth control pills may be difficult to obtain overseas. When possible, take a sufficient supply from home. International Planned Parenthood (www.ippf.org) provides information on contraceptive methods available worldwide.

Condoms are better than nothing, but generally they are inferior to other types of birth control in terms of pregnancy prevention. However, condoms markedly reduce the risk of acquiring sexually-transmitted infections (STIs), so using condoms in addition to another form of birth control is optimal.

Women taking oral contraceptives are at elevated risk of deep venous thrombosis (DVT) and pulmonary embolism (PE)—that is, blood clots in the legs and lungs. This risk is potentially increased further still by traveling to high altitudes (more than 18,000 feet [5,500 meters]). Hence women traveling to high altitudes (e.g., the summit of Tanzania's Mount Kilimanjaro at 19,341 feet [5,895 meters]) should consider stopping the birth control pill prior to the trek and utilizing an alternate method of birth control.

Contraception Q&A

Q I'm overseas for two years. How do I ensure an uninterrupted supply of my birth control pills?

A Obtaining your exact brand of birth control pills while abroad may be problematic. Try to start your time abroad with a one-year supply. Some insurance companies will pay for up to twelve months of pills; some will request a physician's letter. At the end of one year, your best options are either (1) traveling home to get another year's worth or (2) utilizing a family member or friend as a drug mule to bring a year's worth to you. In my experience, mailing medications, either via the post office or a private company such as FedEx, often doesn't work—medications can be held up at Customs or go missing.

Emergency Contraception

About eight in one hundred women of childbearing age will become pregnant after having sex once without birth control during the second or third week of their menstrual cycle. Women of childbearing years not on regular contraception should consider traveling with emergency (post-intercourse) contraception. Options include progestin only, ulipristal acetate, and combined estrogen plus progestin pills.

PROGESTIN ONLY

- levonorgestrel 1.5 mg (e.g., Plan B One-Step in the US)
- Available in the US without prescription
- *Instructions:* one tablet by mouth as soon as possible after unprotected intercourse—the sooner the better
- To be taken within seventy-two hours of intercourse
- Potential side effects include menstrual irregularities, nausea, abdominal pain, fatigue, headache, vomiting, breast tenderness, and diarrhea. In general, progestin emergency contraception has fewer side effects than combined estrogen plus progestin pills.

ULIPRISTAL ACETATE

- ella in the US; ellaONE in Europe
- Prescription required in the US
- *Instructions:* single 30 mg tablet taken once; can be taken up to five days after unprotected sex
- May be more effective for overweight or obese women
- More effective than Plan B One-Step in preventing pregnancy if four or five days have elapsed since intercourse

COMBINED ESTROGEN PLUS PROGESTIN PILLS

- Prescription required
- *Instructions:* pills taken as soon as possible after unprotected intercourse, and again twelve hours later; number of pills depends on the brand
- *Side effects:* About half of women using combined emergency contraception have nausea; about one in five vomits. If you vomit within one hour of taking a pill, repeat that dose again.

The aforementioned emergency contraceptives may be difficult to obtain in low-resource settings. Bringing these from a high-income nation is best.

Although emergency contraception can be taken for up to five days after unprotected intercourse, the sooner it's taken, the higher the odds that it'll prevent pregnancy. Safe abortion services are absent in much of the world.

HIV Post-Exposure Prophylaxis

Those at risk for acquiring HIV infection after an acute exposure (e.g., sex during which the condom broke, sharing needles, sexual assault) should consider taking a course of HIV post-exposure prophylaxis (PEP) medications, which will markedly lower the odds of becoming infected with HIV.

HIV PEP ADULT DOSING SCHEDULE

Truvada (300 mg tenofovir + 200 mg emtricitabine): one tablet per day

Isentress (raltegravir): 400 mg tablet twice per day

Both taken for twenty-eight days.

Timing: HIV PEP must be started within three days of the at-risk exposure—the sooner the better.

Vaginal Infections

Common vaginal infections include yeast infections and bacterial vaginosis (BV). The risk of vaginal yeast infections is increased by the use of antibiotics, including doxycycline taken for malaria prevention. Vaginal yeast infections are characterized by white, clumpy, cottage cheese–like discharge and itching. Treatment is either an oral medication (e.g., fluconazole [Diflucan] tablets, 150 mg once) or intravaginal suppository or cream (e.g., miconazole [Monistat 7], available in the US without a prescription: one applicator full once per day for seven days). Many women find the oral treatment more convenient.

Another common vaginal infection is bacterial vaginosis (BV). This commonly causes a grayish discharge with a fishy odor. The treatment is metronidazole (Flagyl) 500 mg twice per day for seven days, or metronidazole gel 0.75%, one full applicator intravaginally once per day for five days; or clindamycin cream 2%, one full applicator intravaginally once per day at bedtime for seven days.

If initial treatment doesn't cause symptoms to resolve, seeing a medical provider for an exam and laboratory testing is a good idea. The aforementioned medications for vaginal yeast infection and bacterial vaginosis won't treat STIs such as chlamydia and gonorrhea.

OBTAINING MEDICATIONS FOR AS-NEEDED CONDITIONS

If you are prone to bladder infections or vaginal yeast infections, it is reasonable to ask your pre-travel provider for prescriptions for medications to treat these conditions so that you can take them on an as-needed basis while traveling.

Bladder Infections

Most people are not able to self-diagnose most medical problems with accuracy, but bladder infections in women are an exception. Research shows that women who think they have a bladder infection (commonly referred to as a urinary tract infection [UTI]) are usually correct.

Usual bladder infection symptoms are burning with urination, urinary frequency, and an ongoing urge to urinate. Predisposing factors include more frequent sex and dehydration.

Treatment: Options include nitrofurantoin (immediate-release form: 50–100 mg four times per day for five to seven days; extended release form: 100 mg [Macrobid] twice/day for five to seven days) and trimethoprim-sulfamethoxazole (one tablet twice per day for three days). In 2016 the US Food and Drug Administration (FDA) advised that ciprofloxacin (Cipro), and other drugs in its category (fluoroquinolones), commonly used in the past for bladder infections, no longer be used if a different antibiotic is available.

If left untreated, a bladder infection can ascend to become a kidney infection (pyelonephritis). This is a more serious infection. Symptoms include fever and back pain. Those with fever and back pain, whether or not burning with urination is present, should seek medical evaluation.

Probiotics

One area for which probiotic supplements have proven benefit is in the prevention of antibiotic-associated diarrhea. If you're taking an antibiotic for any reason (e.g., doxycycline for malaria prevention, or nitrofurantoin for a bladder infection, or azithromycin for travelers' diarrhea) taking a probiotic concomitantly will reduce the risk of that antibiotic causing diarrhea.

The research supporting other benefits—reducing risk of travelers' diarrhea or vaginal infections—is scanty.

The Pregnant Traveler

Pregnant women can travel to most destinations, but a few caveats are in order. Often women find the second trimester—between weeks 13 and 26 of pregnancy—to be the most comfortable during which to travel.

Live immunizations are avoided during pregnancy. These include measles, mumps, rubella, oral typhoid fever, yellow fever, oral polio, bacille Calmette-Guerin (BCG for TB), varicella (chickenpox), intra-nasal influenza, Zostavax and Vaxchora.

Although traveling in the reduced oxygen environment of a jet (equivalent to 6,000–8,000 feet [1,830 to 2,440 meters] of elevation) is not harmful to either the fetus or pregnant woman, it is said to be inconvenient for all concerned to give birth on a jet, hence travel late in pregnancy (after thirty-six weeks) is ideally avoided. Airlines have different policies regarding flying while pregnant: Many require a physician's note to fly after thirty-six weeks; some require a physician's note to fly after twenty-eight weeks.

Pregnant women are at elevated risk for deep venous thrombosis (DVT) and pulmonary embolism (PE); prolonged sitting, as on a jet or in a car, can exacerbate this risk. Pregnant women on jets should ambulate frequently; women traveling by auto should limit travel to six hours per day, stopping every one to two hours to walk for ten minutes or so. Remaining well-hydrated may also reduce risk. Similarly, I'd advise holding off on high-altitude travel while pregnant.

The flu vaccine (by injection, not intranasal) is safe to receive in pregnancy. So is Tdap (tetanus, diphtheria, pertussis [whooping cough]). Taking azithromycin to treat travelers' diarrhea also is thought to be safe during pregnancy.

Regarding malaria prevention, the antimalarial medication mefloquine is approved for all three trimesters of pregnancy. Given that malaria tends to be more severe in pregnant women, those traveling to areas endemic for malaria should take an appropriate medication.

Women who are infected with dengue fever during pregnancy can transmit the infection to their fetus, resulting in premature birth, low birth weight, or stillbirth. Personal protection measures—applying repellent to exposed skin, applying permethrin to clothing, sleeping under a mosquito net, wearing long sleeves and pants (see chapter 3)—markedly reduce risk. These measures reduce risk not only of dengue fever but also malaria, Zika, chikungunya, and other insect-borne infections. DEET should be avoided in the first trimester of pregnancy but is safe to use during the second and third trimesters, and it is safe to use while breastfeeding. The safety of picaridin, PMD, and IR3535 during pregnancy and breastfeeding have not been established.

Many medications are to be avoided during pregnancy. Discuss any medications you might take with your medical provider.

Pregnant women, at any stage of pregnancy, should not scuba dive. Diving while pregnant has the potential to increase the risk of birth defects and miscarriage. Snorkeling poses no risk related to pregnancy.

Purchasing emergency medical evacuation insurance prior to travel is a good idea.

Zika

Zika, a viral illness transmitted by mosquitoes—and, more rarely, by sex—is now endemic in essentially every country in Central America, South America, the Caribbean, many countries in Africa, and South and Southeast Asia. Infection during pregnancy with Zika virus can cause a plethora of birth defects in the fetus, including microcephaly, a devastating defect in which the fetus has a small head and an underdeveloped brain. The risk of the fetus acquiring birth defects appears to be highest when infected during the first trimester, but it is present for all of pregnancy.

Symptoms of infection with Zika include fever, rash, headache, joint pain, muscle pain, and conjunctivitis (red eyes). Many infections are asymptomatic. Both symptomatic and asymptomatic infections in pregnant women can result in birth defects.

Pregnant women should avoid travel to Zika-endemic countries. If travel to Zika-endemic countries cannot be avoided, pregnant travelers should be diligent regarding the personal protection measures previously listed. Non-pregnant, sexually active women of child-bearing years should use highly reliable birth control.

Breastfeeding

Sterilizing bottles and mixing up powdered formula is a hassle; nursing is more convenient, plus it's better for babies. Nursing babies do not need water supplementation, even in hot climates.

Most medications are secreted in breast milk; many should be avoided during pregnancy. The following are good resources regarding the safety of medications during breastfeeding:
- *CDC Yellow Book* (Health Information for International Travelers): chapter on travel and breastfeeding

- American Academy of Pediatrics: *Medications and Breastfeeding: Tips for Giving Accurate Information to Mothers*
- National Library of Sciences LactMed

The antimalarials mefloquine and chloroquine can be taken by nursing mothers. Malarone can be taken by mothers nursing infants weighting more than 11 pounds (5 kilograms). These antimalarials are excreted in breast milk but not in sufficient quantities to be protective for the infant; hence, infants in at-risk areas should also take an appropriate antimalarial.

Breastfeeding women and their infants should be immunized per routine schedules.

Should a woman who is breastfeeding develop travelers' diarrhea, she should continue breastfeeding—the infection is not transmitted to her infant—and increase her intake of liquids.

THE RELATIVE IMMUNOSUPPRESSION OF PREGNANCY

A pregnant woman experiences changes in her immune system; this phenomenon is known as the relative immunosuppression of pregnancy. The purpose of this may be to avoid reacting to the father's genetic material present in the fetus.

The downside of these changes is that many infections are more serious in pregnant women. A pregnant woman with influenza is more likely to get pneumonia relative to women who are not pregnant, and both malaria and dengue fever are more lethal in pregnant women.

Hence it's particularly important, for both a pregnant woman and her fetus, that she be immunized appropriately (including influenza). She also should take an antimalarial medication when appropriate.

Women Travelers Q&A

Q Are women and men at equal risk for travel-related illnesses and injury?

A No. Women are at higher risk for travelers' diarrhea, post-travelers' diarrhea, irritable bowel syndrome (IBS), upper respiratory infections, urinary tract infections, psychological stress, and adverse reactions to medications.

Women are at lower risk of illnesses with fever (including malaria), sexually transmitted infections, noninfectious issues such as cardiovascular disease, acute mountain sickness, illnesses requiring hospitalization, and trauma including road traffic accidents.

Women are more likely than men to obtain pre-travel medical advice.

Men

The Bottom Line

All causes of violent death and most causes of nonviolent death among international travelers are more common in men, particularly young men. Smart choices mitigate risk.

MEN AGES 18 to 25 have a two- to threefold elevated risk of death while visiting low-income countries, relative to their risk at home, due to what we might term "young male behavior." Young men, as a group, are less risk averse than other travelers. Putting this more bluntly, they do a lot of stupid stuff.

Young men are more likely, relative to the average traveler, to use recreational drugs, drink, drink and drive, drink and drive and crash, drink and swim, drink and swim and drown, drink and socialize, drink and acquire sexually transmitted infections (STIs), and otherwise do themselves bodily harm. Further exacerbating this risk, men are less likely than women to obtain pre-travel advice from a medical professional. Many texts on travel medicine contain chapters on women travelers, but none, to my knowledge, has a chapter on male travelers or, in particular, young male travelers. Perhaps this is an oversight.

Road Traffic Accidents

About half of medical evacuations back to the US are due to injuries sustained in road traffic accidents. Study after study shows that men—particularly young men—are more likely to be injured or killed in these accidents.

One misconception that travelers may harbor is that it's okay to engage in a certain practice because that's the way it's done there. The traveler may be tempted to join locals on the roof of a bus or in the back of an open truck. But these informal locations are extremely dangerous for the locals, as well as for the traveler who joins them. High-income nations have low rates of death and injury from road traffic accidents for a variety of reasons; many pertain to certain high-risk behaviors having been outlawed.

Every year road traffic injuries kill more than 1.2 million people and cause 20 million to 50 million nonfatal injuries. The Association for Safe International Road Travel (ASIRT) was founded by Rochelle Sobel in 1995 after her son Aron Sobel, a fourth-year medical student, was killed in a bus crash in Turkey at age 25. ASIRT's mission is to promote global road safety through education and advocacy. The organization's website lists a wide array of information and strategies to reduce risk. For example, the Road Travel Report on Peru states, with accuracy, "Drivers usually ignore the few traffic signals that exist."

Your control is only partial; you can't do anything about many factors, such as road conditions. However, you can make a number of choices to reduce your risk:

- Don't rent a motorcycle, and don't ride on the back of one. For taxis, use cars, not motorcycles or motor scooters. Imagine yourself going through an intersection and being hit from the side by a car going, say, forty miles per hour. If you're in a car, wearing a seat belt, you're going to get banged up, but long term you're probably going to be okay. If you're on a motorcycle, maybe you'll be killed or paralyzed. It's not worth the perceived convenience, savings, or adventure. If you do ride a motorcycle, wear a helmet.

- Use seat belts whenever possible.
- Avoid roads at night and during bad weather.
- Never travel by road in rural areas after dark. Vehicles are poorly maintained; roads are bad; drivers are worse.
- Don't drink and drive.
- As a pedestrian or cyclist, do not wear any kind of earbuds or headphones. You want to be able to hear traffic and warnings.

Road safety is discussed in further detail in chapter 12.

Drowning

After road traffic accidents, drowning is the most common cause of death of young travelers. More men than women drown. Risk reduction is not complex:

- Learn to swim.
- Don't go into the water without a personal flotation device (PFD) unless you know how to swim. In riskier situations like surfing, kayaking, rafting, or sailing, wear a PFD even if you are an expert swimmer: You can't swim if you've been knocked unconscious.
- Be cognizant of riptides; know how to swim out of one.
- Don't go into the water after drinking or using recreational drugs.
- Don't dive. Enter any body of water feet first.
- Swim with a buddy.

Violent Crime

Yes, for this one too, men are at higher risk. Every big city has districts that are high-crime. Check with locals regarding high-risk areas to avoid. Hotel staff are usually helpful on this topic. Also heed the following:

- Don't wear or carry expensive stuff. Dress down.
- Limit travel at night, especially if you are drinking.

- Travel with a companion or in a group.
- If you're robbed, don't resist. Give everything to the crook.

CHILI TRUCK EPIPHANY

Some years ago I floated a stretch of the Rio Usumacinta, which forms a portion of the border between Mexico and Guatemala, in a dugout canoe with a buddy to see the Maya ruins at Yaxchilan. Afterward, trying to return to a town, I stood at the edge of a dirt road by the river and stuck out my thumb. A truck loaded high with bags of chilies stopped for me. The cab of the truck was already stuffed with people. I asked the truck driver if I could ride in the back of the truck, and he said sure. I climbed to the top of the mound of sacks of chilies. It was a pleasant perch. This was late May, the hottest, most humid season, and after all the sweaty days in the dugout, the motion of the truck created a welcome breeze. Insects, dense on the river, seemed to be leaving me alone.

After some hours of reverie—I grew distracted—in an instant a big tree branch, fully half a foot thick, whizzed inches from my head. Smaller branches and leaves swept the sunglasses from my face. I wasn't hurt, but I did have a realization. The truck driver had not given me permission to climb into the back of his truck because it was safe. He'd said okay because I'd asked, and rides were then scarce at the Mexico–Guatemala border, and he was trying to be helpful. Had I been sitting a scootch to one side, that fat branch would have brained me.

I no longer hitchhike.

I no longer ride in the back of trucks.

Suicide

Suicide is more common in men. If you're experiencing an exacerbation of depression, isolating yourself in a foreign country can make you feel even worse. Depression and other psychiatric issues can be helped by counseling and medications, but these may be harder to locate abroad.

When you're depressed, talking with someone—a friend, a professional, or both—is invariably a good idea. The blog Together We Are Strong lists telephone helplines in more than fifty countries around the world (http://togetherweare-strong.tumblr.com/helpline).

Note: The antimalarial mefloquine should not be used by people with a history of depression, anxiety, or other psychiatric disorders; it can cause an exacerbation of symptoms.

Drug Overdose

Drug overdose is more common in men. It's particularly disadvantageous to overdose in low-income nations because, if you survive, medical support will be minimal.

Some people travel for the express purpose of trying a new psychogenic drug, such as ayahuasca, a brew prepared from a particular vine, utilized by some indigenous peoples of the Amazon basin. This is ill advised. My thought is that if trying new hallucinogens or other recreational drugs is your thing, limit experimentation to the high-income nations, where you will have adequate medical support should it be needed.

Psychiatric emergencies are one of the most common reasons that tourists and other international travelers require emergent medical evacuation. A significant number of those evacuated for psychiatric reasons have used recreational drugs, which may have contributed to the need to evacuate.

Additionally, many foreign countries have draconian drug laws, with sentences ranging from lengthy prison terms to the death penalty. Potential sentences for drug offense convictions in Malaysia, Singapore, Saudi Arabia, and Iran include caning, flogging, lashing, or whipping. In Singapore, if you are found to possess three or more grams of morphine, you will get the death penalty.

If you have a drug habit—opiates or other—talk with your doctor. In addition, regular attendance at a support group such as Narcotics Anonymous correlates to remaining drug free. Narcotics Anonymous groups meet in countries around the world, including Mexico, Peru, India, and Thailand. See www.na.org/meetingsearch. And, of course, never share needles.

Sexually Transmitted Infections

Sexually transmitted infections (STIs) are more common in men. Condoms. Condoms. Condoms. They are fully legal to transport through Customs. They should be latex condoms, manufactured in a high-income nation.

Some men travel with the intent of paying for sex. My advice: Don't do it. If the ethics of sex tourism aren't sufficient inducement to refrain from paying for sex, be aware that STIs, including HIV, are markedly more common in commercial sex workers than in the general population. Additionally, the areas where this industry thrives are also common sites for tourists to be robbed.

If you do have a high-risk exposure, consider starting a twenty-eight-day course of HIV post-exposure prophylaxis (PEP), which will markedly lower the odds of becoming infected with HIV.

HIV PEP ADULT DOSING SCHEDULE
Truvada (300 mg tenofovir + 200 mg emtricitabine): one tablet
    per day
Isentress (raltegravir): 400 mg tablet twice per day
Both taken for twenty-eight days.
Timing: HIV PEP must be started within three days of the at-risk
    exposure—the sooner the better.

Older Men

Although men become more risk averse as they age, they continue to die abroad at a higher rate than do women. At a given age, men are more likely than women to have cardiac issues, including heart attacks (myocardial infarctions), while traveling. A markedly higher level of exertion while traveling relative to your baseline at home is unwise. If trekking or climbing is involved in your trip, pre-travel training is smart.

High altitude can exacerbate cardiac or pulmonary conditions such as angina or chronic obstructive pulmonary disease (COPD). If your itinerary contains a high-altitude destination (e.g., Quito, Ecuador: 9,350 feet [2,850 meters]; Cusco, Peru: 11,152 feet [3,399 meters]; the summit of Mount Kilimanjaro, Tanzania: 19,341 feet [5,895 meters]), run your itinerary and planned activities past your physician. Older men may take longer to acclimate to high altitude. Consider adding a few days to your itinerary upon arrival at high altitude to just hang out and acclimatize. Seek medical attention for symptoms such as chest pain or shortness of breath unrelieved by rest.

Many people have more frequent sex while on holiday, and many men use a medication for erectile dysfunction (ED) such as sildenafil (Viagra), tadalafil (Cialis), or vardenafil (Levitra). In addition to the side effects of headache, facial flushing, nasal congestion, diarrhea, and backache, these medications cause a drop in blood pressure. Men who take nitrates (e.g., nitroglycerine, isosorbide) should not take one of these ED drugs, as they can experience a dangerously low drop in blood pressure.

The FDA urges caution regarding these medications in patients with a history of heart attack, stroke, heart arrhythmia, congestive heart failure, unstable angina, low blood pressure, and uncontrolled high blood pressure (over 170/110). These drugs are available in several strengths. Men with cardiovascular disease should start at low to moderate doses, then adjust the dose depending on results.

If you're going to use one of the ED drugs, it's better to obtain it in a high-income nation—quality control of medications purchased in low-income nations may be suboptimal.

Men Travelers Q&A

Q Avoid motorcycles? But I'm traveling with the specific intent to ride a motorcycle.

A It's your call—I'll only reiterate that it's a risky activity. Plus, keep in mind that should you sustain an injury, medical facilities are often substandard. If you plan to ride a motorcycle, it's all the more important that you purchase emergency evacuation insurance. And remember to take a helmet with you.

Q Instead of packing condoms, can I buy them at my destination?

A Condoms manufactured in low-income nations may be substandard and may leak or be more prone to breakage. And, as with medications and brand-name fashion accessories, consumers need to be aware of counterfeit products—same brand name, markedly lower quality.

Condoms should be latex and manufactured in a high-income nation. The stakes are high. Every year an estimated five hundred million people become infected with chlamydia, gonorrhea, syphilis, or trichomoniasis. In 2016, an estimated 1.8 million people became infected with HIV. Use of condoms markedly lowers risk of transmission of all STIs.

Q What about tattoos?

A Think before you ink. A design that strikes you as fundamentally emblematic of your being may, in twenty or forty years, lead to what is termed *tattoo regret*. One study showed that almost one-third of people with tattoos wish they hadn't gotten them.

Avoid getting tattoos in low-income nations, where inks may be substandard and needles may not be sterile, which could lead to infection with HIV, hepatitis B, hepatitis C, and a number of other pathogens.

Q I take Adderall for ADHD. Are there any issues related to taking that overseas?

A Maybe. Adderall (amphetamine and dextroamphetamine) and Ritalin (methylphenidate) are amphetamines, and are illegal in some countries, including Japan. Some countries want a doctor's letter or a copy of the original prescription for certain drugs. A nation's embassy in the US is often a good source regarding laws and regulations. See additional sources of information of traveling with medications in the Resources for Global Travelers section at the end of this guide. (The male-to-female ratio for ADHD is approximately 4:1.)

Q I like to seek out the local nude beach and sunbathe.

A Careful—misery may ensue when the sun shines where the sun don't shine. Your nether regions can burn surprisingly quickly. And insect bites—*aiee!* First, apply sunblock, wait fifteen minutes or so, then apply insect repellent. Shower before intercourse.

LGBTQ Travelers

The Bottom Line

Many countries are inclusive regarding lesbian, gay, bisexual, transgender, and queer (LGBTQ) travelers, many are not. Research regarding local laws and attitudes prior to your trip is prudent.

Pack copies of family- and health-related documents, including marriage license, durable power of attorney, and adoption forms.

THE GLOBAL TREND is going in the right direction. South Africa and Argentina legalized same-sex marriage in 2006 and 2010, respectively. In 2015, Luxembourg's prime minister, Xavier Bettel, became Europe's first leader to marry a same-sex partner while in office. Uruguay has become a leader in transgender rights; a law passed in 2009 allows people to change their name and legal gender on official documents to match their gender identity.

However, while most high-income and many low-income nations have become increasingly inclusive of LGBTQ persons in recent years, consensual same-sex sexual relations remain illegal in more than seventy nations. For example, in Uganda, under the Penal Code Act, "carnal knowledge against the order of nature" between males carries the potential punishment of life imprisonment. Female homosexuality is illegal as well.

Choosing a Destination

LGBTQ travelers should research the attitudes and policies of their destination prior to travel. Western Europe is generally inclusive; Saharan and sub-Saharan Africa are often not. Depending on local attitudes, it may be prudent to not reveal your sexual orientation. In Muslim-majority countries, open displays of affection, regardless of your orientation, are to be avoided. Transgender travelers may face unique challenges, ranging from airport screenings to bathroom issues.

The International Gay and Lesbian Travel Association website (www.iglta.org) lists LGBTQ travel businesses and destinations. Damron (www.damron.com), founded in 1964, publishes both men's and women's guides to gay travel, as well as a number of gay-oriented city guides. The *Spartacus International Gay Guide*, published annually, is another travel guide. In addition, many guidebook series, including Lonely Planet and Footprint, routinely include sections on gay and lesbian travelers.

LAWS

A helpful website for determining laws regarding LGBTQ persons is Equaldex (www.equaldex.com), a collaborative knowledge base that lists LGBTQ rights by country and region. In addition to detailing laws regarding consensual sexual activity between individuals of the same sex, it also lists laws regarding marriage, changing gender, adoption, employment, discrimination, housing discrimination, military service, donating blood, age of consent, and conversion therapy.

At the US Department of State's Country Information page (https://travel.state.gov/content/travel/en/international-travel/International-Travel-Country-Information-Pages.html), click "Local

Laws & Special Circumstances" for any country to see a summary of laws pertaining to LGBTQ travelers.

Safety

Prudent planning and decisions reduce risk.

POLICE AND ENTRAPMENT

In some countries in which homosexual activity is illegal, police and other authorities monitor websites, mobile apps, and meeting places. In such places LGBTQ travelers should keep an eye out for entrapment campaigns. Travelers should be cautious when connecting with the local community. Criminals may attempt to extort LGBTQ foreigners. Also, some vacation resorts or LGBTQ areas can be markedly segregated, such that surrounding neighborhoods can be much less accepting.

CRUISING

If you plan on visiting a cruising area, or using a dating app to meet someone:
- Inform a friend and/or have a friend in the vicinity.
- Meet in a public place, such as a restaurant. Avoid being picked up or dropped off by the person being met.
- Limit the personal information that you share. Crooks sometimes exploit the generally trusting and relaxed nature of the gay community.
- Your alcohol and/or drug consumption should be minimal or none. You want to retain your good judgment.

Health

Threats to health can be minimized by smart decisions.

If you do hook up, always engage in safe sex. Outbreaks of sexually transmitted illnesses, including syphilis, have been linked to using phone apps such as Grindr and Craigslist to find sex partners. If you do have a high-risk exposure (e.g., a condom breaks), consider a twenty-eight-day course of HIV post-exposure prophylaxis (PEP) to reduce risk—see chapter 12 for details.

If you are taking a medication such as emtricitabine/tenofovir (Truvada) for HIV pre-exposure prophylaxis (PrEP), continue to take it and continue to be screened for sexually transmitted infections (STIs), including HIV, every three months. If you are HIV-positive and taking routine medications for that (highly active antiretroviral therapy [HAART], to suppress HIV replication), don't stop taking medications while abroad. Stopping these meds is linked to serious illness and death.

GENDER CONFIRMATION SURGERY

To save money, some people travel outside of high-income nations for gender confirmation surgery. It can be difficult to determine what standards of training and practice a surgeon in a low- or middle-income income nation must meet, as well as what recourse you have if something goes wrong. Globally the quality of care is uneven and may be substandard in some areas, there is often a paucity of post-surgical care and complications may lead to a longer stay abroad than initially planned and considerable additional expense. Avoid holiday packages—recovery from surgery can take weeks to months, and you are unlikely to enjoy vacation-related activities.

MENTAL HEALTH

Being in the closet after living openly at home is stressful. It may be disconcerting not to be able to hold your partner's hand while strolling down the street. Your sense of vulnerability and isolation may be heightened by the knowledge that your sexuality is considered criminal.

The LGBTQ traveler may have difficulty finding sensitive and affirming care abroad. Keep in mind that discrimination against LGBTQ persons is associated with a higher rate of mental health disorders, substance abuse, and suicide relative to the non-LGBTQ population. If you feel in need of support, most mental health issues can be helped by counseling and/or medications. Talking with someone—counselor, friend, other—is helpful. The Trevor Project is a private organization that provides crisis intervention and suicide prevention services to LGBTQ people ages thirteen to twenty-four. Via its website (www.thetrevorproject.org) you can connect with counselors by phone, instant messaging, or texting.

Other Practical Considerations

Before you leave for your trip, consider how your paperwork lines up with your family configuration. It may be important to have marriage and/or adoption documents not only for border crossings but also for securing hotel accommodations and hospital access in the case of medical emergencies. Alternately, disclosing less relationship status information may be safer in some circumstances, as many countries do not legally recognize same-sex marriage. If you have a power of attorney document or healthcare proxy form, pack those; married travelers should bring a copy of their marriage license. (A Seattle acquaintance recently encountered cultural misunderstanding when a physician in Sri Lanka was baffled that both she and her wife were the mother of their ill child.)

UPDATE YOUR PASSPORT

Currently, the only two options for gender on US passports are male and female. If your name or gender presentation has changed, you should update your passport. Information on this process can be found at the US Department of State website (www.state.gov). The US State Department website also provides some helpful information at its LGBTI Travel Information site (https://travel.state.gov /content/passports/en/go/lgbt.html).

TSA AND AIRPORT SECURITY ABROAD

Advanced imaging technology may lead to a pat down, which can be very upsetting for transgender travelers. If travelers cannot, or choose not, to be screened by advanced imaging technology or a walk-through metal detector, they may request a pat-down procedure instead. Pat downs will be done by an officer "of the same gender as you present yourself" per Transportation Security Administration (TSA) policy. Screening can be performed in a private screening area to which travelers may take their carry-on luggage, with a companion of the traveler's choosing. Travelers will not be asked to remove or lift any item of clothing. Travelers may ask to speak with a supervisor at any time during screening.

See the TSA Transgender Passenger page at https://www.tsa.gov /transgender-passengers. Also helpful is the National Center for Transgender Equality travel page: https://transequality.org/issues/travel.

The airport security procedures of many countries are more complex than those utilized in the US, and they may entail vehicle searches, bomb-sniffing dogs, and multiple security checkpoints.

Also, anything you pack may be examined at airport screening, drawing unwanted scrutiny and, potentially, additional screening.

TRAVEL INSURANCE

Consider purchasing travel insurance (see chapter 1). Some travel insurance companies sell plans specifically tailored to LGBTQ travelers. You should confirm that your insurance plan covers all family members who are traveling.

Children

The Bottom Line

- One of the most enriching experiences that parents can share with their children is to take them to a foreign country.
- With few exceptions, a child can go anywhere an adult can go.
- As with adults, prudent precautions (booster seats/car seats/seat belts, immunizations, and a medication to prevent malaria, if needed) will minimize risk.

I AM A big proponent of taking kids on the road. Children who do not travel tend to think that their particular corner of the world is representative; children who travel will realize that most who live in high-income nations are wealthy and fortunate. Children of immigrants (and recall that all of us who live in the US and Canada, with the exception of Native Americans, are relatively recent immigrants) will benefit from visiting the land of their forebears and learning about their heritage firsthand. Selfishly, another reason to take kids abroad is that they open doors. In much of the world, you will not be fascinating by dint of having originated from a faraway land, but everyone loves a cute kid. If you travel with a child, people will talk with you, open up to you, and come to your aid much more readily than if you are traveling by yourself or only in the company of other adults.

Jet Travel

Parents who take children on long jet rides with no planned entertainment for their kids will regret it. For the very young—ages 2 to 3—consider wrapping some favorite and familiar toys and bringing them aboard the jet. It's two pleasures in one: first the joy of unwrapping something, then a favorite toy! (Do not try this on adults.) Also, an ample supply of water and snacks is a must. Remember that departure times may be delayed, connections may be missed. Take more diapers and snacks than you anticipate needing. Imagine yourself backpacking with your young one(s) for twenty-four hours. What might you need? It's a pain to haul all this stuff around, but it would be worse to run out of diapers on a prolonged delay on the tarmac.

Most airlines will not allow a child under age 5 to travel unattended by an adult. If traveling with a small baby, make your reservations as early as possible and try to reserve seats in the first row of your section. A bassinet is often built into the dividers between sections. Most US domestic flights do not require the purchase of a ticket for children under age 2 (who then sit on a parent's lap). However, most international flights require tickets for all children. Fortunately, many international carriers do not charge full price for children's tickets, and they may charge as little as 10% of the cost of an adult ticket. Travel by air is safe for children of all ages, including newborns.

Vigilance

If you are traveling with a toddler, get down on your hands and knees at each new hotel room and crawl about and see what your wee one might attempt to knock over, stick a finger into, or eat.

Bring plastic outlet covers. They're cheap and weigh almost nothing, although those built for standard US outlets may not fit foreign outlets.

TWO BOYS, TWO WEEKS, GUATEMALA

In summer 2006 my wife and I took our two boys, then ages 5 and 7, to Guatemala for two weeks. We spent a week in Panajachel and a week in Antigua, touring coffee and macadamia nut plantations and visiting nearby villages.

Our boys enjoyed our relaxed rules regarding soda pop (primarily Fanta Orange). Daily they asked us to buy them machetes and daily we said no. We took them to a *brujo* (sorcerer) ceremony on a hilltop outside Chichicastenango. We thought they might be alarmed when the *brujo*, a thirtyish man in jeans and a T-shirt, pulled the head off a live chicken, but they were nonplussed and thought it fascinating that the headless corpse kicked its legs for some time.

At the end of the two weeks, both boys wanted to stay longer. However, the elements with which they bonded were not those that we had anticipated.

NATE AND HENRY'S LIST OF OUR FAVORITE
THINGS ABOUT GUATEMALA:

5. People ride in the backs of trucks.

4. Machetes for sale everywhere.

3. Rain so hard the streets were rivers.

2. Fanta Orange.

1. They execute chickens.

Water Safety

Drowning is most common around the world in children under age 5, in both boys and girls. A study that looked at sixty-eight British children who drowned abroad between 1996 and 2003 found that 71% of deaths occurred in swimming pools, most of which were hotel pools.

STRATEGIES TO REDUCE RISK
- Bring personal flotation devices (PFDs) and have your children wear them when they're in or around water. Assume that your destination will not be able to supply these.
- Maintain close parental vigilance.
- Do not trust a child's life to another child.
- If you are choosing between hotels with pools, try to stay at one with a climb-resistant fence (one that is at least 4 feet [1.2 meters] high).
- Avoid swimming lessons for children before the fourth birth-day. A loss of normal wariness around water may more than counterbalance the benefits of being able to swim (although some authorities support swim lessons in children ages 1–3).
- Teach children to ask permission to go near water.
- If a child is missing, check the water first.

Motion Sickness

Children are all over the map in their response to motion: Some are unbothered while riding in a small boat in a stormy sea, and some lose their breakfast during a two-minute drive on a straight and smooth road. To reduce motion sickness while on a jet, sitting a child next to a window, facing forward, and avoiding big preflight meals may be of some help. Some kids do better during night flights, when they can sleep.

Over-the-counter drugs that help some children include Benadryl (diphenhydramine), Dramamine (dimenhydrinate), and Antivert (meclizine).

- *Benadryl (diphenhydramine):* The dose is proportionate to weight: a 50-pound (23 kilograms) child would receive 25 mg every six to eight hours. Benadryl is not for use in those under age 1. It is available in a liquid preparation. Maximum dose is 50 mg.
- *Dramamine (dimenhydrinate):* Children ages 2 to 6 should be given ¼ to ½ of a chewable 50 mg tablet every six to eight hours, not exceeding 1 to 1½ tablets in twenty-four hours. Children ages 6 to 12 should be given ½ to 1 chewable 50 mg tablet every six to eight hours, not exceeding 3 tablets in twenty-four hours.
- *Antivert (meclizine):* This drug is for those over age 12; the dose is 25–50 mg, thirty to sixty minutes prior to travel. Repeat if needed every four to six hours, not exceeding 150 mg per day.

Usually diphenhydramine, dimenhydrinate, and meclizine help kids with mild to moderate symptoms of motion sickness. For severe symptoms not controlled by the above drugs in children over age 2, the use of promethazine (dispensed by prescription only) can help. The Transderm-Scop (scopolamine) patch, also available by prescription only, is approved only for those over age 12. (Also see chapter 13.)

Vaccinations

ROUTINE VACCINATIONS

As with adults, the most important vaccines are not the travel or exotic ones but, rather, domestic ones. Recall that many diseases that are rare in high-income nations, such as hepatitis A and B, and measles, are common in lower-income nations. Your child should be current for vaccinations for hepatitis A and B, diphtheria, pertussis, tetanus, Haemophilus influenzae type b, polio, measles, mumps, rubella, varicella (chickenpox), pneumococcal disease, rotavirus, meningococcal disease, influenza, and human papilloma virus (HPV).

The advised pediatric vaccine schedule is available online at several websites. One way to access it is to search online for *pediatric vaccination schedule*. Sites that post the current schedule include the CDC, AAFP (American Academy of Family Practice), and AAP (American Academy of Pediatrics).

Children between ages 6 and 12 months traveling to areas endemic for measles (including most of sub-Saharan Africa) should receive a single dose of MMR vaccine, which does not "count"—that is, they then later need to be revaccinated via the usual schedule (one dose of MMR between ages 12 to 15 months, and a second dose at least four weeks later). Children between ages 1 and 4 who have had a single dose of MMR vaccine should have a second dose, at least four weeks after the first. This is a "countable" dose and does not need to be repeated at ages 4 to 6.

REQUIRED VACCINATIONS

As with adults, only two vaccines are required in pediatric travelers to some destinations. Travelers to many countries in tropical South America or tropical Africa are required to be vaccinated for yellow fever; this vaccine is given only to children over age 9 months. (Yellow fever vaccine *may* be given to infants 6 to 8 months, but they have an increased risk of significant adverse side effects; most authorities advise holding off on vaccinating with yellow fever prior to 9 months.)

Children traveling to Mecca in Saudi Arabia for the Hajj or Umrah are required to be vaccinated for meningococcal meningitis. This must be administered at least ten days and no more than three years prior to entry for the polysaccharide vaccine and no more than eight years prior to entry for the conjugate vaccine (Menactra, Menveo). The CDC recommends revaccination with conjugate vaccine after five years for those at ongoing risk. (*Note:* The Hajj is a religious duty for adults, not children.) The vaccine is also advised for those traveling to the "meningitis belt" of Africa (see map 3 in chapter 2) and for those who will be staying in crowded living quarters, such as college freshmen living in dorms. Minimum ages: Menactra, 9 months; Menveo, 2 months. Current standard schedule in the US for children: first dose of conjugate vaccine at 11 to 12 years, second dose at age 16.

THINGS TO ADD TO YOUR TRAVEL KIT IF TRAVELING WITH CHILDREN

- *Car seat or booster seat.* These can be scarce outside of high-income nations. If you have a child of car-seat or booster-seat age, take one along. This is the most important precaution you can take for your child. Consider, at the end of your trip, leaving it behind for use by others.
- *A lead test kit.* Paint may contain lead. Even in the US, lead-based paint for use in housing was not banned until 1978. A lead test kit is cheap (about US $6) and only weighs an ounce or two. You drip a bit of the test kit solution onto whatever you're curious about; a color change indicates the presence of lead. If your hotel or apartment has lead paint—move! Consuming even a small amount of chips of paint with lead can lead to symptoms in children.
- *Over-the-counter (OTC) medications.* I suggest that you carry several over-the-counter medications: ibuprofen (Advil, Motrin), diphenhydramine (Benadryl), hydrocortisone 1% cream, and an antifungal cream such as terbinafine (Lamisil). Also, assume your young one will tumble and scrape a knee, so take some sort of antiseptic wash (although soap and water are almost as good) and antibiotic ointment such as Polysporin or Neosporin. Antiseptic hand wipes confer some reduction in risk of food-borne and water-borne infections.
- *Whistle.* Consider, if hiking with children, giving each child a whistle to use in case he or she becomes lost.

Hepatitis A

All international travelers age 1 and above should receive vaccination for hepatitis A, which is spread by contaminated food and water. Children older than 1 year should receive the usual vaccine: two immunizations separated by at least six months. The CDC recommends that travelers under age 1 going to at-risk regions (essentially all low- and middle-income nations) receive a single dose of IG (gamma globulin) for the prevention of hepatitis A; however, many pre-travel providers, realizing that symptoms of hepatitis A are minimal or absent in the very young, advise forgoing this.

Influenza

Influenza is one of the most common infectious diseases seen in international travelers. Vaccination for influenza is recommended for almost everyone over age 6 months, with the exception being if the child has had a prior life-threatening reaction to a flu vaccine or has a severe allergy to any component of the vaccine.

Typhoid fever

Typhoid fever, spread by contaminated food and beverages, is present worldwide outside of high-income nations; risk to travelers is greatest in South Asia (the Indian subcontinent). It is particularly important for children who will be spending a long time (i.e., more than one month) at at-risk destinations, or who will be in remote or particularly rustic or rural environs (e.g., small villages or camping), to receive this vaccine. Typhoid fever has been contracted by even short-stay visitors. As with adults, the vaccine comes in two forms: a shot (approved down to age 2, which provides protection for two years); and four pills (approved for use in children above age 6; protection is good for five years). The four pills require refrigeration and are taken on an empty stomach: one pill every other day.

Rabies

Rabies vaccine is not routinely recommended for a child traveling on a short-term vacation to a routine tourist destination, such as a beach in Mexico or the Caribbean. However, it should be considered for children on itineraries with higher risk (rural stay, village stay, prolonged stay, children of missionaries or other expatriate workers). The primary vaccine series consists of three doses, given over twenty-one to twenty-eight days. Most people do not require booster doses.

Teaching is important. Many children have a natural tendency to pet dogs, cats, and other animals. However, outside of high-income nations this places children at increased risk for a panoply of diseases, including rabies.

Recall that the fatality rate for rabies, once the first symptoms develop, is 100%. After any bite or other potential exposure to mammal spit (including playing with a dead bat), (1) wash the wound with soap and copious water, then (2) see a physician for treatment whether or not your child has had the pre-exposure vaccine series.

Japanese Encephalitis

See the discussion under adult vaccinations in chapter 2. Vaccination for Japanese encephalitis is not advised for children under age 2 months.

Preventing Travelers' Diarrhea in Children

The feeding option that carries the lowest risk of travelers' diarrhea in infants is nursing. For older children, the same precautions that adults are advised to follow may be of some benefit. Children should not take preventative antibiotics, Pepto-Bismol, or other drugs that contain salicylates.

Treatment of travelers' diarrhea in children is different from that for adults. For openers, the entire flouroquinolone class (e.g., ciprofloxacin

[Cipro] or levofloxacin [Levaquin]) should be avoided in those under age 18. For children, azithromycin is a good choice for all destinations. One regimen is 10 mg/kg once per day for three days.

Anti-motility drugs such as loperamide (Imodium) should be avoided in children under age 6.

Parents should have a low threshold for seeking medical care for children with diarrhea. Fever, bloody stools, significant abdominal pain, and failure to improve one to two days after beginning antibiotics are all reasons to have the child see a physician.

Small children are at risk of dehydration from travelers' diarrhea. There are several commercial preparations of oral rehydration therapy (ORT) salts that are packaged in foil wrappers; the parents mix the powder with sterile water. Alternatively, the solution is easy to produce on your own: Add one-half level teaspoon of salt and six level teaspoons of sugar to a liter of clean water. Consider adding half a cup of pasteurized juice or a single-serving packet of powdered flavoring, such as Tang, to improve the taste.

SUGAR IN THE MEDICAL KIT?

I learned a good low-budget trick when I attended a tropical medicine course in Lima. For significant skin wounds—large abrasions and such—ordinary white sugar as purchased from the grocery store makes an excellent topical antibiotic. It is not only bacteriostatic (keeps bacteria from growing) but bactericidal (kills bacteria on contact) due to the osmotic pressure it exerts (imagine salt on snails). It's cheap, it's easily available. Its downside is that it tends to make a mess during dressing changes, and in tropical climates ants will materialize in a moment if you leave any on the floor. In a pinch, though— if you do not have an antibiotic ointment—reach for the sugar bowl.

Traveling with Children with Allergies

Food allergies are common: 1 in 13 children is allergic to at least one food. For unknown reasons the proportion of children with food allergies is increasing worldwide. When traveling with the child with food allergies, a few precautions are in order.

- When you book your ticket you can ask your airline to serve your child food without whatever he or she is allergic to, but in my experience, more often than not, this is not relayed to the flight staff, who do not have anything other than standard fare. It's probably best to carry sufficient allergen-free food for the flight(s).
- Pick your restaurants with care. Even in high-income nations, wait staff will often have no idea what the food contains. If your child's allergic reaction has been severe (swelling, difficulty breathing), it might be best to forgo restaurants entirely, and eat only what you buy yourself at the grocery store.
- Realize that food labels may be substandard—not fully accurate—outside of high-income nations.
- As with other medicines, do not place your EpiPens and diphenhydramine (Benadryl) in checked luggage; place them in your carry-on bag.
- Prior to your trip, or on arrival in a new town, learn where the medical center is. Learn how to say *allergy* and *hospital* in the language of the country you are in.

I would not forgo international travel for a child with food allergies, but heightened vigilance is necessary. Food Allergy Research and Education (FARE) is a nonprofit with considerable helpful information for the international traveler with food allergies, including a Food Allergy & Anaphylaxis Emergency Care Plan on its website: www.foodallergy.org.

The Adolescent Traveler

Adolescence is a period of discovering boundaries and pushing limits. I think it's a great idea to take an adolescent abroad, but there may be a disconnect between adolescents' still-developing judgment and their suddenly expanded range of options, such that they can do significant harm to themselves should they make poor decisions.

Regardless of your policy on piercings and tattoos, you must stress to your adolescent children that they must not get a piercing or tattoo outside of high-income nations for reasons that I discuss in chapter 18.

Parents should discuss safe sex with teens. This is particularly important before trips during which teens will have less supervision.

Post-Travel Screening for Children

TUBERCULOSIS (TB)

If your child spends a long duration—years—in an at-risk destination (and tuberculosis is common worldwide outside of high-income nations), getting a test for latent TB—either a skin test (a PPD) or a blood test—a minimum of eight weeks after return is a good idea. (In children under 5 years the skin test is preferred.) Similarly, should a child who has spent time in an at-risk destination develop a cough that lasts for more than three weeks, testing is indicated.

SCHISTOSOMIASIS

Any child who has fresh water exposure in an area endemic for schistosomiasis (bilharzia)—such as a lake in Africa—should have screening for this illness. This screening is a blood test performed a minimum of six to eight weeks after the most recent potential exposure.

For those returning after lengthy stays abroad, consider a stool exam, even in those without symptoms.

Kids Abroad Q&A

Q Are there some itineraries for which we should leave the kids at home?
A You bet.

High altitude: There is no reason to take a child to high altitude. Studies have not been performed on the effects of high altitude on children. It would not be ethical to march a thousand children up to 20,000 feet (6,100 meters) and see how they do. The travel medicine community is split on the issue of children's sensitivity to altitude illness. Some providers feel kids are about as sensitive to altitude illness as are adults; some think they are a little more prone. The problem is that the signs of acute mountain sickness in children—irritability, fussiness, fatigue—are identical to the early signs of more serious problems, including high-altitude pulmonary edema and high-altitude cerebral edema, which are also identical to the signs of a crabby or tired kid who is having no problem whatsoever with altitude. With preverbal children, it's impossible to tell if they only want a nap or if they are feeling short of breath or confused. I would advise that you leave your children with relatives or a sitter at low altitude.

Those with Down syndrome are more susceptible to high-altitude pulmonary edema.

In 2001 a committee of twenty-five experts on high-altitude illness published a consensus statement which concluded, "Drug prophylaxis [e.g., Diamox—generic name: acetazolamide—commonly used by adults] to aid acclimatization in childhood should usually be avoided." The authors also pointed out the following:

- There are no data about safe absolute altitudes for ascent in children.
- The risk of acute altitude illness is for ascents above about 8,200 feet (2,500 meters), particularly sleeping above that elevation.
- Intercurrent illness might increase the risk of altitude illness.
- Effects of long-term (weeks) exposure to altitude hypoxia on overall growth and brain and cardiopulmonary development are unknown.

Security risks: If for some reason you are going somewhere with a high risk of civil turmoil or crime, leave the wee ones at home.

Yellow fever: Babies under age 9 months should not receive the vaccine for yellow fever; hence, they should avoid travel to regions in tropical South America and tropical Africa that are endemic for yellow fever. (Babies under age 9 months have a risk of encephalitis, a life-threatening condition, if they receive this vaccine.)

Q What about taking a child to an area with malaria?

A Although malaria may be more severe in children than in adults, I think that as long as the child takes an appropriate antimalarial drug, and parents are conscientious in their use of personal protection measures (DEET or picaridin to exposed skin, permethrin to clothes, bed net) for the child, children should not be barred from regions in which malaria is present. DEET is safe for children over age 2 months, although concentrations of DEET over 30% are to be avoided in children. Picaridin should not be used in babies under age 2 months; oil of lemon eucalyptus (OLE) should not be used in children under age 3.

Both Malarone (approved for use in children over 11 pounds [5 kilograms]) and mefloquine (no lower limit on age) are approved for children. The psychiatric side effects of mefloquine appear to occur less commonly in children. Doxycycline may be used in children age 8 and older. Chloroquine and hydroxychloroquine have no lower age limit. Information regarding doses are available at www.cdc.gov.

Store all medications, including antimalarials, on a high shelf, in childproof containers. Consuming an overdose of antimalarial medication can cause severe illness or death in small children.

Q **What's the deal with ear infections and jet travel?**

A Worries about jet travel causing eardrums of children with ear infections or head colds to rupture have been shown to be unfounded. However, ear pain in children with upper respiratory infections can certainly worsen during air travel. (The air inside a jet is not pressurized to the equivalent of sea level but, rather, to about 6,000 to 8,000 feet [1,830 to 2,440 meters].) Premedication with acetaminophen (Tylenol) or ibuprofen (Motrin) will help minimize discomfort and crying.

Q **What about taking a car seat and using it on the jet?**

A The Federal Aviation Administration (FAA) "strongly recommends" but does not require the use of a car seat (they don't call it a car seat [or jet seat]; they call it a "child restraint system" [CRS]) for children weighing less than forty pounds (18 kilograms).

All car seats manufactured after January 1, 1981, have been found to be acceptable for jet travel. Your CRS should have the statement "This restraint is certified for use in motor vehicles and aircraft" printed on it. You may be required to check, as baggage, any car seats without this statement printed on them.

11

Travelers with Chronic Medical Problems

The Bottom Line

Many people with chronic illnesses travel to low- and middle-income nations every year; the vast majority return no worse for their time abroad. Certain preparations and precautions may need to be undertaken, but most people with most illnesses should not limit their travel abroad due to their state of health.

MOST PEOPLE WITH most medical problems can visit most destinations, but additional planning may be necessary. Travelers with chronic medical problems should seek pre-travel care at least two months prior to departure. In addition to seeing a pre-travel provider, travelers with chronic medical conditions should run their planned itineraries and activities past their usual physicians. As a general rule, symptoms—angina, shortness of breath, seizures, and so on—should be well controlled at the traveler's nation of origin before considering international travel.

All prescription medications should remain in the packaging in which they are dispensed from the pharmacy, with the names of the traveler and physician clearly legible. Similarly, all nonprescription medications should remain in the original packaging. Medications should be transported in carry-on, not checked, luggage. One strategy is for travelers to carry a full supply of medication in their carry-on, then an additional 50% to 100% of surplus medication in checked luggage, in case of theft. Check with the US embassy or consulate of the country you're visiting to ensure that there are no restrictions concerning your medications. Some nations ban the import of certain medications, particularly narcotics and psychotropic medications (e.g., Adderall [amphetamine and dextroamphetamine]).

Travelers with medical conditions that might result in loss of consciousness (e.g., seizures, diabetes, coronary artery disease) should wear medical alert bracelets that list medical problems, medications, and allergies. The MedicAlert Foundation (www.medicalert.com) is a nonprofit organization that supplies medical alert bracelets and serves as a repository for medical information. Their TravelPlus program is specifically designed for travelers.

It is particularly important for travelers with chronic medical conditions to have both medical insurance and emergency medical evacuation insurance. (See the discussion of this topic in chapter 1.) Additionally, trip cancellation insurance, in case of unexpected illness, can save you money.

A listing of medical clinics abroad is available from the International Association for Medical Assistance to Travelers (www.iamat .org). See Resources for International Travelers.

The US Department of Homeland Security's Transportation Security Administration (TSA) Cares Helpline (toll free: 855-787-2227) provides information regarding preparation for airport security screening with respect to specific medical problems or disabilities.

Diabetes Mellitus

Some people think that insulin, like milk, spoils rapidly if not refrigerated, but in fact it's pretty hardy stuff. If you can keep it under 82°F

(28°C), it will last four weeks, so for most short-term trips, refrigeration is not necessary. Then again, if you plan to leave it in your car in the desert in the summer, store it with a cold pack. The insulin preparation lispro (Humalog) is convenient when traveling as it is particularly fast and short acting; it can be taken at the beginning of a meal, as opposed to regular insulin, which must be taken thirty to forty-five minutes prior to eating.

If you cross five or fewer time zones or travel north to south, you don't need to alter your daily insulin schedule. If you travel through six or more time zones, altering your schedule is necessary. Eastward travel results in a shortened day, and less insulin is needed. Skipping the evening dose when flying eastbound will cause only somewhat elevated glucose, and it may help to prevent you from becoming hypoglycemic. One authority suggests decreasing the total daily dose of insulin by 2% to 4% for every hour of time change during eastward flights, as well as increasing the total daily dose by the same amounts for westward flights. More frequent than usual determinations of glucose—every four to six hours—may be appropriate during travel, even if you don't check your glucose that frequently at home.

Travelers who control their diabetes with oral medications only, and not insulin, do not require additional doses and should take their medication according to local time. Try to avoid skipping meals.

Also, realize that mealtimes outside high-income nations do not occur with clockwork regularity. Buses break down, drivers get lost, waiters may return with food several hours after you place your order. Carrying a supply of something sweet is smart. Insulin-dependent diabetics should consider carrying glucagon, particularly if their glucose levels are unstable.

Those who attempt to maintain their usual level of good control of their glucose values while traveling across time zones run the risk of hypoglycemia. It's probably better to accept glucose values that are somewhat elevated on travel days.

The website of the American Diabetes Association (www.diabetes .org) is a source of information regarding airline policy for carrying medications and supplies for diabetes, as are the individual airline carriers. Laws regarding prescription drugs vary country to country; the International Diabetes Federation (www.idf.org) is a valuable source of information regarding this. Learning to say "I have diabetes" and "Sugar or orange juice, please" in the language of your destination is prudent.

Other sources of information regarding diabetes and international travel are www.diabetes.org/pre-diabetes/travel/when-you-travel.jsp and www.diabetesmonitor.com; the latter lists examples of specific insulin regimens.

Chronic Bronchitis or Emphysema

Airplanes do not pressurize to the equivalent of sea level but to about 6,000 to 8,000 feet (1,830 to 2,440 meters). Ask your physician if he or she advises that you use oxygen when you fly. If you require oxygen at home while at rest, you should not attempt flight without oxygen. You should notify the airlines well in advance of your planned flights, as most US carriers will not allow you to bring your oxygen on board; you must use their supply. Discuss your itinerary with your physician prior to your trip. Depending on the severity of your bronchitis or emphysema, your physician may advise you to avoid high-altitude destinations.

Bad smog may preferentially affect those with chronic bronchitis or emphysema (see chapter 12). Most big cities in low- and middle-income nations have heavily polluted air. Again, discuss your travel plans with your physician. If your chronic bronchitis or emphysema is severe, you may want to minimize your stay in such cities.

Coronary Artery Disease

As with people with chronic bronchitis or emphysema, people with coronary artery disease (CAD) or a history of myocardial infarction (MI, or heart attack) are at increased risk at high altitudes or in heavily polluted air. It's all about oxygen: CAD causes the heart to receive a diminished supply of blood and hence a diminished supply of oxygen; an MI is caused when the supply of blood is so low that part of the heart muscle dies. Both elevated altitude and heavily polluted air further reduce the ability of blood to carry oxygen. Again, run your travel plans by your physician.

If you tend to develop angina with prolonged walking, you should inform the airline that you require wheelchair assistance when you reserve your ticket. If given sufficient notice, airlines can provide this, including gate-to-gate transport at connecting airports.

Travelers with CAD should be able to walk for a hundred yards and climb twelve steps before they fly. People who have had an MI should avoid travel by air for at least one month afterward. Those with unstable angina, or symptoms at rest, should avoid travel by air altogether.

Travelers should pack an abundant supply of their medications; some cardiac drugs may not have exact equivalents in foreign countries.

It is prudent for travelers with CAD and those who have had myocardial infarctions to pack a copy of their most recent EKG for comparison purposes, should emergency care be required. Additionally, a summary letter from your physician, including results of stress tests (treadmills), cardiac catheterizations, and other studies, should be carried.

A German study of 200 travelers with pacemakers and 148 travelers with implantable cardioverter-defibrillators found that none was affected by airport metal detectors. A pre-travel check with your cardiologist to make certain that the device is working properly, and that battery life is sufficient, is advised. (See the Chronic Bronchitis or Emphysema section in this chapter if you require oxygen.)

HIV/AIDS

For people with HIV/AIDS, the best measure of the strength of the immune system is a recent CD4 count (peripheral count of CD4+

lymphocytes). Additionally, it is helpful to determine a viral load; those with a CD4 count of less than 200 (or CD4 less than 15%) with high viral load are at significant risk of new infections.

If your CD4 count is above 200, your physician may recommend that you receive live vaccines. If your CD4 count is below 200, you should avoid live vaccines (measles, mumps, rubella, oral typhoid, yellow fever, varicella [chickenpox], shingles [Zostavax is live; Shingrix is not], cholera [Vaxchora] and intranasal influenza), due to a theoretical possibility of developing illness from the attenuated virus or bacteria. Some authorities recommend that people with HIV/AIDS receive vaccines three to six months after initiation of highly active antiretroviral therapy (HAART).

People who are HIV-positive should be up to date on their pneumococcal, diphtheria–tetanus, hepatitis B, and influenza vaccines. Non-live vaccines, including hepatitis A, hepatitis B, polio, and meningococcus, should be given as they would be to non-HIV-positive travelers. The injection form of typhoid vaccine, which is killed, should be given instead of the oral (live) vaccine.

Yellow fever vaccine, which is also live, should be considered by HIV-positive travelers going to an endemic region if their immunosuppression is minimal or absent, as indicated by a CD4 count over 200. Some authorities state that only travelers with a CD4 count over 400 should receive vaccination for yellow fever.

Note: Those who are HIV-positive should never receive bacille Calmette-Guerin vaccine (BCG), which is for prevention of tuberculosis. BCG is not routinely advised for travelers from the US.

Food- and water-borne illness may be more severe in people with HIV/AIDS, and following safe food guidelines (see chapter 4) is prudent. Taking an antibiotic on a regular basis for the prevention of diarrhea is controversial. Some pre-travel providers advise a preventative medication to reduce the risk of travelers' diarrhea in their travelers with HIV/AIDS. An advantage of rifaximin (marketed under the brand name Xifaxan in the US) for this purpose is that it is not absorbed in significant amounts; hence risk of drug interactions is extremely low. However, unfortunately, rifaximin is currently extremely expensive.

Malaria can be more severe in people with HIV/AIDS. Travelers to areas endemic for malaria should adhere to standard malaria prophylactic medication guidelines and be diligent in their use of personal protection measures, including DEET and permethrin. There are multiple potential drug interactions between antimalarials and medications used by people with HIV/AIDS; these should be discussed with your physician and/or pharmacist. Antimalarials should be started well in advance of international travel so that the traveler can be monitored for drug interactions and adverse drug effects. If you are on antiviral medications, you should be on a stable regimen for at least eight weeks prior to international travel; this allows time to identify medication side effects.

Some travelers with HIV/AIDS take a drug "holiday" from their usual HIV medication regimen during their travels, but this is ill-advised; interrupting antiviral medications has been linked to increased risk of illness and death.

Check HIV/AIDS entry restrictions in the "Entry, Exit, and Visa Requirements" section. Another helpful resource is the Global Database on HIV-related travel and residence restrictions (www.hivtravel .org/Default.aspx?pageId=142).

Chronic Renal Failure

Hemodialysis is available around the world but should be scheduled several months in advance. The largest database of dialysis centers is online at www.globaldialysis.com; it lists over 16,800 dialysis centers in 161 countries. The National Kidney Foundation (www .kidney.org) can facilitate scheduling. The Society for Accessible Travel and Hospitality (www.sath.org) lists information on travel and cruise boat companies that organize trips specifically designed for travelers on dialysis.

People on dialysis require higher-than-standard doses of vaccine for hepatitis B. The effect of dialysis on most antimalarials is unknown; however, dialysis does not affect blood concentrations of mefloquine.

Multiple Sclerosis

Although there have been case reports of onset or exacerbation of multiple sclerosis (MS) following vaccinations, multiple large, well-controlled studies have failed to identify a link between vaccinations and short-term exacerbations. However, there is significant evidence that relapses of MS are linked to antecedent infections, including upper respiratory infections. This suggests that travelers with MS should receive vaccination for infectious illnesses for which their travel places them at significant risk.

Immune Suppression and Immunizations

TYPE OF IMMUNE SUPPRESSION	CAUTIONS/SUGGESTIONS
Recipient of kidney, heart, lung, or liver transplant	Avoid international travel for one year post-transplant. Get pneumococcal, meningococcal, and Hib (*Haemophilus influenzae* type b) vaccines. Get hepatitis B and influenza vaccines pre-transplant.
Hematologic malignancies (e.g., leukemia)	No live virus vaccines* for three months after last therapy. Get pneumococcal and Hib (*Haemophilus influenzae* type b) vaccines, ideally two weeks before suppressive therapy; also IPV (polio), influenza, and diphtheria, tetanus, and pertussis (DTaP); also measles-mumps-rubella (MMR) and varicella (chickenpox) if not severely immunosuppressed.
Congenital immune disorders	No live vaccines.+

TYPE OF IMMUNE SUPPRESSION	CAUTIONS/SUGGESTIONS *(cont.)*
Drug-induced immunosuppression (e.g., chronic steroid use of over 20 mg prednisone or its equivalent/day)	No live vaccines.[+] Vaccinate one month or more after last dose of steroid.
Hyposplenism (having had spleen removed, or having a nonfunctioning spleen due to sickle cell anemia or other cause)	Get pneumococcal, meningococcal, Hib (*Haemophilus influenzae* type b), and influenza vaccines.
Multiple sclerosis	No change in standard vaccine practices.

[*] Live virus vaccines: measles, mumps, rubella, yellow fever, varicella (chickenpox), zoster (shingles [Zostavax is live, Shingrix is not]), influenza (intranasal, not via injection), and rotavirus.

[+] Live vaccines: measles, mumps, rubella, oral typhoid, yellow fever, BCG (for TB), varicella (chickenpox), influenza (intranasal, not via injection), rotavirus, cholera (Vaxchora), Zostavax.

Source: This table is adapted from "Challenging Scenarios in a Travel Clinic: Advising the Complex Traveler," by Kathryn N. Suh and Maria D. Meleno, *Infectious Disease Clinics of North America*, vol. 18, number 1 (March 2005).

Travelers with Chronic Illness Q&A

Q I'm HIV-positive, and my CD4 count is below 200. I'm going to a country that requires visitors to have immunization for yellow fever (a live vaccine). What should I do?

A Ask your pre-travel provider to fill out the waiver section of your yellow vaccine card (International Certificate of Vaccination or Prophylaxis), stating that you are unable to receive that vaccine for medical reasons. (I wouldn't list the exact medical reason that precludes the vaccine—this could cause delays or other complications at Customs.) And then realize that you are not protected for a disease that, although not common in tourists, can be catastrophic even in those with intact immune systems. If you decide to go, anti-insect personal protection measures (DEET to skin, permethrin to clothes, sleeping under a net) are all the more important.

Q I'm HIV-positive, and I'm significantly immunocompromised (my CD4 count is under 200). Does international travel put me at higher risk of illness than others?

A Yes.

Q Does that mean I should cancel my plans to travel to low-income nations?

A That's your call.

Q Come on! Give me a little guidance here.

A I'm serious. It's a complex topic, and there's no one right answer. International travel to high-income nations (e.g., western Europe) puts you at increased risk for head colds and influenza; these tend to be more severe in people who are immunocompromised.

Travel in low- and middle-income nations puts you at increased risk for, among other illnesses, infections that cause diarrhea, and again these tend to be more severe in those with immunosuppression. Compounding this, medical care may be remote and/or substandard. So the threat to health is significant—but so is the reward. To see the game parks of Africa, or the Mayan pyramids of Chiapas and Central America, or the temples of southeast Asia are wondrous experiences. The risk is high, the reward is high. It's complex. It's your call.

Q Whatever happened to "doctor's orders"?

A We don't give orders anymore. We share information and make recommendations.

Q What's your recommendation?

A My recommendation is that you make the call.

Q How can I find a good medical provider while traveling abroad?

A See the discussion of about the International Association for Medical Assistance to Travelers (IAMAT) in Resources for International Travelers.

Activities and Environs

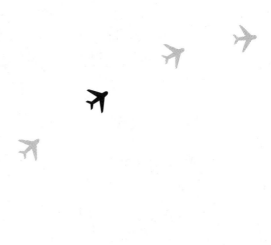

12

Cities and Social Situations

The Bottom Line

- The most common cause of death of young, fit travelers is road traffic injuries.
- Seat belts are good.
- Don't ride in the back of a truck or on the roof of a bus.
- Stay off the roads at night.
- Don't ride motorcycles, motor scooters, or mopeds.
- If you have sex with a new partner, using condoms is smart. Not using condoms is dumb.

EVEN IF YOUR ultimate destination is rural and remote, you almost always must transit through a big city en route. Most travelers to the game parks of East Africa fly into Nairobi, population four million; most travelers to the beaches of southern Thailand fly into Bangkok, population eight million; most travelers set on trekking to Machu Picchu in Peru fly into Lima, population ten million. Surviving the megacity is requisite for arriving at your final and rustic destination.

I would not try to dissuade you from visiting big cities in low-income nations. Poor big cities are wonderful and terrible at the same time; they contain the best and the worst of humanity. But—and this is my key point—preparation and particular strategies can minimize your chance of something untoward occurring while in the metropolis.

When most people think about threats to the health of international travelers, their first thought is infectious disease: malaria, yellow fever, cholera. However, studies about the causes of death of those who foray from affluent countries to low-income nations consistently show that infectious diseases—all infectious diseases, including pneumonia, malaria, yellow fever, cholera, kidney infections, typhoid fever—account for only about 1% to 2% of tourist deaths. About half the deaths are due to heart attacks and strokes; these occur primarily in the elderly.

So what is the most common cause of death in young healthy travelers? Simple: road traffic accidents, including car crashes, motorcycle crashes, and bus crashes (or being a pedestrian who is hit by a motor vehicle). Road traffic accidents are the number one cause of the demise of nonelderly international travelers. Even a 10% reduction in deaths in international travelers due to motor vehicle crashes would save more lives than would total elimination of deaths in international travelers from all infectious diseases.

Road Traffic Accidents

Travel by car has become markedly more safe in recent years in high-income nations. In the US, fatalities per one hundred million miles traveled in a vehicle have dropped from 18 in the 1920s, to 5 in the 1960s, to 1.1 in the past decade. This precipitous drop is due to many factors, including enhanced vehicle safety features (seat belts, air bags, other), helmet laws, more stringent drunk driving laws, and improved road design.

Travel by automobile is markedly more dangerous in low-income countries. Low-income countries account for only about 1% of the world's automobiles, but 16% of the world fatalities from motor vehicles occur in those countries.

Road Fatalities per 100,000 Inhabitants Per Year (2015 Data)

Europe	9.3
Americas	15.9
Africa	26.6

The statistics are even more dramatic for annual road fatalities per 100,000 motor vehicles.

Annual Road Fatalities per 100,000 Motor Vehicles (2015 Data)

Europe	19
Americas	33
Africa	574
UK	5
US	13
China	104
India	130
Uganda	837
Togo	3,653
Somalia	4,480
Ethiopia	4,984
Guinea	9,462

Source: Adapted from World Health Organisation (WHO), ed. (2015). WHO Report 2015, Violence and Injury Prevention. Data Tables A2, A10. Geneva: WHO. www.who.int/violence_injury_prevention/road _safety_status/2015/GSRRS2015_data/en

Although deaths from many infectious causes, including malaria and measles, are declining, deaths from motor vehicle injuries in low- and middle-income nations are sharply increasing. In 2011, deaths from motor vehicles caused 2.2% of global deaths and ranked as the ninth-leading cause of death. By 2030 this is projected to increase to 3.6% of deaths, ranking as the fourth-leading cause of death. This rapid increase is due in large part to the growth of car ownership in middle-income nations.

The pattern of fatalities differs between high- and low-income countries. In the US, more than 60% of road traffic accident fatalities occur in drivers; in low-income nations, fewer than 10% of fatalities occur in drivers. In low- and middle-income nations, most traffic deaths are of vulnerable road users, including pedestrians and bicyclists. Urban pedestrians alone account for about 65% of auto-related deaths in poor countries.

There are many, many reasons that road traffic accidents are more common in low- and middle-income nations. The roads are bad, cars are in poor condition, people do not follow the laws, the laws are not enforced, people ride in creative places such as the roofs of buses and the backs of open trucks, kids don't ride in car seats, vehicles do not have seat belts, and people do not use them if they do.

Drunk driving is also an issue. The percentage of drivers with blood alcohol levels higher than 80 mg/dl, indicating impairment, has been found to be 0.4% in Denmark; 3.4% in France; and 21% in Accra, the capital of Ghana. Alarmingly, 4% of bus drivers and 8% of truck drivers in Ghana were found to have blood alcohol levels above the level of impairment.

Compounding the high rate of accidents, no formal emergency medical system is established in most low-income countries. If you crash your car, you do not call 911—there is no operator standing by. You hitchhike, taxi, walk, or crawl to the nearest medical facility, which, if you are in a rural area, may consist of little more than a well-intentioned village healer. Research shows that your odds of dying from a life-threatening injury are markedly higher in a low-income nation— in one study odds were 36%, as opposed to 6% in a high-income nation.

Not surprisingly, this translates into a higher rate of death via road traffic accidents in tourists. Male travelers between ages 15 and 44 have a two to three times higher rate of death in low-income nations as compared with the same age group in high-income nations.

- *Most important:* Seat belts are good. There is no single intervention in a motor vehicle that will raise your odds of surviving a crash as dramatically as will wearing a seat belt. A combined lap and shoulder belt is best, but using a lap belt alone yields significant benefits.
- Avoid renting anything motorized and two-wheeled. If you do, wear a helmet. If you ride a bike, wear a helmet. Do not ride as a passenger without a helmet.
- Avoid road travel at night, especially in regions where drivers keep their headlights off at night. Someone told me this is because of a belief that using headlights will run the battery down. With these unilluminated yet high-speed cars and trucks, livestock on the road, pedestrians on the road, and wrecked vehicles on the road, it makes sense to limit your road time to daylight hours.
- Avoid riding in the back of an open truck, including taxis in which passengers sit on benches along the bed of a semicovered pickup truck (e.g., *songthaew* in Thailand), or on the roof of a bus, or in or on other "informal" riding locations. If you are in the back of a truck, or on the roof of a bus, and that truck or bus suddenly turns or stops, you become a projectile—that is, you become airborne until you strike something sufficiently solid to stop you, such as a tree. The tree will do well; you will do poorly. Ride inside.
- Don't be macho. So some guy cuts you off? Let him. So some car passes you even though you are driving the superior vehicle? So what? Derive your sense of self-worth from some other avenue than besting other motorists.
- When you're a pedestrian, don't attempt to multitask: Don't attempt to read your smartphone or guidebook while walking. Sidewalks may be uneven; deep holes may appear unexpectedly. Don't walk around wearing headphones or with earbuds in your ears: You need to be able to hear vehicles, sirens, and other sounds. And when you step into a street, remember what your parents told you when you were five: Look both ways.

Winston Churchill fought in six wars and was taken as a prisoner of war in South Africa. And where did the sole traumatic injury of his life occur? New York City. In 1931, near New York City's Central Park, Churchill looked right to check for traffic as he stepped into the street and was struck by a taxi. He sustained a scalp laceration down to his skull and two fractured ribs, and was hospitalized for a week. Even on one-way roads, even if you do not hear a car: Look both ways before stepping into the street. Similarly, if you are driving in a country in which cars drive on the side of the road opposite to the side you're accustomed to, it would not be overkill to place a hand-written note to yourself on the dashboard—Drive on the left!

If you've spent significant time in low-income nations, you will immediately see a problem with my advice. The truth is that many—most?—vehicles in low-income nations do not have seat belts. However, if you find a taxi with a seat belt, ask the driver to come to your hotel the next morning when you think you'll need a taxi. I advise helmets for cyclists—many rental places do not stock them. If you are renting a car in advance, ask the rental agency if all its cars have seat belts. If you plan on renting a bicycle, take a helmet with you. I advise that you do not rent anything motorized and two-wheeled—but if you do, do not even think of starting off without a helmet.

So, what should you do about this high rate of crashes? I've just told you that roads are markedly less safe than those in low-income nations and that road traffic accidents are the number-one killer of nonelderly international travelers. Should you just cross the non-wealthy nations off your itinerary?

Well, it's your call—but here's my take. If you do poorly with shades-of-gray discussions, skip ahead to the next section. My thought is that, in essence, it's worth it. Even taking the high rate of road traffic accidents into account, recall that only 1 in 100,000 international travelers dies abroad. The vast majority of people who travel to low-income nations return home intact and yearning for more international travel. Yes, the roads are more dangerous, but you can tweak the odds in the right direction by following the preceding advice.

Other Causes of Accidents and Trauma

It is not only cars that can do you harm in cities of low-income nations. A few years back I saw a college student with a sinus infection at my clinic. As we chatted, I noted several large healed surgical scars over his left elbow. I asked what had happened, and he said that two years prior he had visited Istanbul, Turkey, and stepped into an old-style cage elevator in an office building. Momentarily distracted, he allowed the cage door to close on his arm. He couldn't free his arm. The elevator then changed floors. He was lucky that his arm wasn't amputated. Take-home message: While abroad, low-level ongoing vigilance is good. Precipices may not be marked, glass doors may not have decals to keep you from walking into them, or you may see a springy diving board over water that is only 4 feet (1.2 meters) deep.

And don't sit under the coconut tree. Think about it: coconuts, gravity, your head. People die every year from being hit on the head by coconuts. Had Sir Isaac Newton been sitting under a coconut tree instead of an apple tree, he would have had no further insights whatsoever. Although not a common cause of death, it takes little effort to lay out your towel outside the drop zone.

Air Pollution

The first attempt to control air pollution occurred in 1306 CE, when England's King Edward I banned the burning of coal in an effort to control the malodorous clouds of coal smoke over London. The ban was not enforced, and London became one of the first cities to suffer from significant air pollution.

The US Environmental Protection Agency terms the six principal air pollutants *criteria air pollutants*; these are carbon monoxide, nitrogen dioxide, ground-level ozone (not to be confused with "good ozone," which is in the stratosphere at six to thirty-one miles [ten to fifty kilometers] above the earth), particulate matter, sulfur dioxide, and lead. Each of these has multiple deleterious effects on health:

- Particulate matter increases the risk of premature death in people with heart or lung disease, worsens asthma, and decreases lung function. It also increases the risk of lung cancer.
- Ozone reduces lung function and can cause throat irritation and coughing; it worsens bronchitis, emphysema, and asthma.
- Carbon monoxide reduces the amount of oxygen that the blood can transport and can exacerbate angina in people with heart disease.
- Nitrogen dioxide (NO_2) can aggravate respiratory diseases, including asthma; long-term exposure elevates risk of

developing asthma and can increase susceptibility to respiratory illnesses.

- Sulfur dioxide (SO2), which is formed by the burning of fossil fuels such as oil and gas, is harmful to the respiratory system; children, the elderly, and those with asthma are particularly susceptible to the effects of SO2.
- Lead adversely affects the nervous system and the kidneys, and it hampers immunity.

You do not need to memorize which cities in low- and middle-income nations have polluted air; it is safe to state that virtually all big cities in low-income nations have crummy air. Globally, 80% of urban areas have air pollution exceeding levels recommended as healthy by the World Health Organization (WHO). Among cities in low- and middle-income countries with population over 100,000 people, 98% have unhealthy air. And the trend is getting worse: Between 2008 and 2013, global air pollution levels rose by 8%.

When I say that low-income nations have crummy air, I do not mean that their air is a little more polluted than air in affluent big cities; I mean that their air is fantastically worse. PM2.5 stands for particulate matter less than 2.5 microns in diameter—a complex mix of floating bits of pollution (both small particles and liquid droplets) that are so tiny that they can lodge deep in the lungs and cause significant health issues.

The US Environmental Protection Agency (EPA) has set a limit for PM2.5 of 12 micrograms per cubic meter. Los Angeles, a city with bad air pollution by US standards, has an average PM2.5 level of 12.6. In November 2017 the air in New Delhi, India, was extremely bad, with PM2.5 levels above 1,000, said to be equivalent to smoking fifty cigarettes per day. In 2018, the WHO issued a report stating that the fourteen cities with the highest $PM_{2.5}$ levels are all in India.

If you're young and fit, breathing bad smog for a few days is unlikely to cause anything worse than stinging eyes, a cough, and a sore chest. However, some people's asthma is made worse by smog.

Particulate Matter (PM$_{2.5}$), Worst Cities (2008–2015)*

LOCATION	MICROGRAMS PER CUBIC METER
1. Zabol, Iran	217
2. Gwalior, India	176
3. Allahabad, India	170
4. Riyadh, Saudi Arabia	156
5. Al Jubail, Saudi Arabia	152
6. Patna, India	149
7. Raipur, India	144
8. Bamenda, Cameroon	132
9. Xingtai, China	123
10. Baoding, China	123
11. Delhi, India	122
12. Ludhiana, India	122
13. Dammam, Saudi Arabia	121
14. Shijiazhuang, China	121
15. Kanpur, India	115

*Most values are more recent than 2013.

The elderly and those with preexisting cardiac or pulmonary conditions can have serious health issues with smog.

Carbon monoxide binds to the hemoglobin in your red blood cells with a much greater affinity than does oxygen. The net result is that your blood is less able to carry oxygen to your body. The carboxyhemoglobin level is that percentage of your red blood cells' hemoglobin that is attached not to oxygen but to carbon monoxide. People with chronic cardiac disease (e.g., coronary artery disease) or pulmonary problems (e.g., chronic bronchitis or emphysema) may develop angina or shortness of breath at a carboxyhemoglobin level of 3% to 4%. Vigorous exercise in a heavily polluted city can raise the carboxyhemoglobin level to 5% within ninety minutes. Additionally, elevated carbon monoxide levels have been shown to increase the rates of hospitalization for people with a history of congestive heart failure. Both long-term and short-term studies have found that a number of constituents of smoggy air, including ozone and particulates, correspond to both hospital admissions and deaths.

Long-term exposure to ozone raises the risk of developing asthma; short-term exposure to ozone causes increased risk of pneumonia and exacerbations of asthma and chronic obstructive pulmonary disease. Of course, as with smoking, long-term exposure to several components of smog will raise your risk of lung and other cancers. However, virtually all of the research that has been done on the health effects of smog have concentrated on long-term residents of polluted regions; our thoughts regarding the effects of air pollution on travelers are based on extrapolation and guesswork.

What does all this mean for the international traveler? People with a history of asthma that has been made worse by air pollution will obviously want to minimize their exposure to polluted cities. In addition, it would be prudent for people with asthma to travel with an additional inhaler, as well as an oral steroid such as prednisone or methylprednisolone (Medrol Dosepak), for as-needed use. Travelers with a history of chronic obstructive pulmonary disease (either chronic bronchitis or emphysema) should carry, in addition to their usual medications, a three-drug "rescue cocktail" for exacerbations, consisting of an additional inhaler, an appropriate antibiotic, and an oral steroid. Travelers with shortness of breath that is not quickly improved with those additional medications should have a very low threshold for seeking medical care.

Prior to travel, elderly travelers may want to consider getting a physical exam that includes stress treadmill and pulmonary function testing. Certainly travelers with known cardiac or pulmonary disease will want to have those conditions under good control prior to their departure. (See chapter 11.)

Travelers with a history of cardiac or pulmonary disease may want to minimize their duration of stay in heavily polluted cities and avoid heavy exercise while residing therein. For some, airport transfer only—one jet to another—may be the wiser option.

Heat Illness

Cities, like mountains, are capable of creating their own weather. Asphalt and concrete absorb light, then reradiate it as infrared radiation, raising the temperature. Termed the *urban heat island effect*, this infrared radiation often raises city temperature 2°F to 10°F. For example, the population of the Phoenix Valley region in Arizona grew more than tenfold between 1944 and 1984, from 150,000 to 1.8 million; during that period, its average summertime lows increased by 8°F. In June 2017, commercial jet flights to Phoenix were cancelled because the extremely hot air—119°F—was too thin to provide adequate lift.

Every year, hundreds of people in the US are killed by heat illness; the elderly are particularly at risk. During the European heat wave in the summer of 2003, more than seventy thouand people died from the effects of the heat. Because of climate change, extreme heat waves are becoming more common. In May 2017, the temperature in Turbat, Pakistan, reached 128.3°F (53.5°C); in June 2017, the Iranian city of Ahvaz saw a temperature of 129.2F (54°C).

Thermoregulation is our bodies' method of keeping us cool in hot places and warm in cool places. Thermoregulation is impaired by a variety of factors, including a number of drugs (e.g., phenothiazines, anticholinergics, diuretics, beta blockers, and alcohol; see the following table).

At rest, our core temperature doesn't vary much: approximately ±0.5°F (±0.3°C) at rest. This increases up to 3.6°F (2°C) in more extreme temperatures while exercising.

Ordinarily, sweat cools us down. It's hot, we sweat, the sweat evaporates, we feel cooler. However, when the humidity is high, sweat does not work: you sweat, it does not evaporate, you do not feel cooler. In high humidity, sweating only leads to fluid loss.

Drugs That Can Impair Thermoregulation and Make You More Susceptible to Heat Illness

CATEGORY	EXAMPLES
Phenothiazines	promethazine (Phenergan)
	prochlorperazine (Compazine)
	chlorpromazine (Thorazine)
Anticholinergics	dicyclomine (Bentyl)
	diphenoxylate and atropine (Lomotil)
	hyoscyamine (Levsin, Levbid)
	scopolamine (Transderm-scop)
	trihexyphenidyl (Artane)
	benztropine (Cogentin)
	diphenhydramine (Benadryl)
Diuretics	hydrochlorothiazide (Microzide)
	chlorthalidone (Hygroton)
Beta blockers	metoprolol (Lopressor)
	propranolol (Inderal)
	atenolol (Tenorim)
Alcoholic beverages	Budweiser

Note: diphenhydramine is both an anticholinergic and an antihistamine.

Over 240 years ago, Scottish physician James Lind wrote that habituation to hot climates leads to a lessened risk to health; this has been borne out by modern research. After several days in a hot climate, core body temperature and heart rate become less elevated, the ability to sweat increases, and the concentration of salt in sweat drops to one-third of what it is in the nonacclimatized; these changes allow you to survive and thrive in a hot environment.

Drinking a lot of fluids is a good idea. Do not rely on thirst to tell you that you need to drink more water. It's really hot, and you've drunk eight liters of water, you haven't had to urinate for six hours, and you feel fine? That means you need to drink more water. Drink water to the point that your urine is close to colorless. Use the marathoner's rule: dark yellow urine = drink more water.

Avoiding the midday sun is smart. In hot environs, you may want to live a crepuscular lifestyle: most active at dawn and dusk. There is wisdom in the Latin American custom of *la siesta*—the afternoon nap.

Sexual Activity

Having sex with a new partner while abroad is not uncommon. In one Spanish study, 19% of international travelers had a new sexual partner while abroad, and only about half used condoms. Alarmingly, a high percentage—3.4%—of those who did not use condoms acquired HIV infection. An Australian study showed that only one in three travelers would *not* have sex with a new partner should an opportunity arise. (I'm not implying that the Australians are particularly randy; I think the figures would be similar for many countries.) Overall, studies show that 5% to 50% of travelers sleep with someone new while abroad.

The likelihood of having a new partner while abroad is higher in men, in those traveling without their usual partner, and with increasing duration of stay. In a study of 1,200 Peace Corps volunteers, 60% had sex with another Peace Corps volunteer, and 39% reported sex with a host country national. Of those who had a new partner while abroad, only 32% used condoms consistently. The typical sex tourist—someone who travels for the express purpose of hiring commercial sex workers—is male, with an average age of 38. A majority do not use condoms.

Not surprisingly, the risk of acquiring HIV is markedly higher while abroad. One UK study showed that the risk of international travelers was three hundred times higher while abroad compared with their at-home risk. The prevalence of HIV in commercial sex workers is twelve-fold that of the general population.

Of course, HIV is only one of many afflictions you can pick up via your sex life. Gonorrhea, chlamydia, herpes, syphilis, venereal warts, and hepatitis B are among the many infections that are sexually transmitted diseases (STDs). (I could go on. Some of the more disturbing photos I have viewed during my study of tropical medicine are photos of men's and women's genitals with a variety of sexually transmitted infections: granuloma inguinale, lymphogranuloma venereum, and chancroid. You do not want a photo of your privates grossing out a group of doctors in training.)

As to whether or not you have a new partner in your sex life while abroad, that's your business. But sleeping with someone new without using a condom is dangerous. People who have a high-risk sexual encounter, or other risk for HIV (sharing needles and works, sexual assault) should consider a course of HIV PEP (post-exposure prophylaxis) to reduce risk of acquiring HIV. This consists of taking a twenty-eight-day course of three medications, tenofovir + emtricitabine (Truvada) and raltegravir (Isentress), which will markedly lower risk. The regimen should only be used in emergency situations, and must be started within seventy-two hours of the exposure—the sooner the better. The US Department of Health and Human Services website, which is supported by the Secretary's Minority AIDS Initiative Fund (SMAIF), has good info on this: https://www.hiv.gov/hiv-basics/hiv-prevention/using-hiv-medication-to-reduce-risk/post-exposure-prophylaxis. The CDC has a helpful PDF on this at https://www.cdc.gov/hiv/pdf/programresources/cdc-hiv-npep-guidelines.pdf.

Women at risk for pregnancy should consider taking a medication to prevent pregnancy within seventy-two hours of unprotected sex. (See chapter 7.)

Crime and Security

Although usually not a health issue per se, crime in many cities in low-income nations, as in many cities in high-income nations, is common. International travelers may be viewed as walking automated teller machines. The math isn't complex: They're poor, you're rich. Do not carry your valuables in a fanny pack (*bum bag* in UK parlance).

These are easy targets for thieves. Carry one if you want, but keep only lunch and trinket money in it. Beware the mustard scam, in which someone sprays something on your clothes, then helps you by wiping it off as they help themselves to whatever they can find in your pockets. If someone points out something on your clothes—keep walking. Some thieves prefer the slash 'n' grab technique, in which the bottom of your bag is slashed with a very sharp knife and the crook grabs whatever falls out.

If malefactors demand your wallet, or anything else on your person, *give it to them*—even if you are personally affronted by your assailant's behavior, even if you are big and strong and they are small. A knife or gun wielded by even a small person can send you to the sphere of heavenly reward sooner than you want to see it.

War, major internal strife, and natural disasters are not spectator events. Countries with significant turmoil should be avoided. Street demonstrations in low-income nations can turn violent with little warning; you should not photograph or join in protests. The US State Department maintains a list of countries for which they have issued travel warnings; this is available on the department's website: http://travel.state.gov/travel/warnings.

Wearing clothes with a military appearance—camouflage-pattern fatigues and such—is unwise in low-income nations, many of which have a history of unwelcome military intervention in their recent past. Travelers dressed in garb reminiscent of armed forces may draw attention from police and security personnel.

Crime and Security Q&A

Q I want to take my laptop computer. Is that a problem?
A Maybe. Unless you need your computer for study or business, consider leaving it at home. Let's look at the pros and cons of keeping your journal on a laptop, as opposed to writing in longhand on a clipboard or in a spiral-bound notebook.

	LAPTOP	CLIPBOARD
Price	Expensive	Cheap
Power needs	Needs electricity	Doesn't need electricity
Adaptor plug	Adaptor plug needed for most low-income destinations	No adaptor plug needed
Affected by sunlight	Useless in bright sunlight	Not hampered by bright sunlight
Potential for theft	High	Near zero
Durability	Can be damaged by humidity or rough handling	Nearly indestructible; not adversely affected by high humidity

I've left my writing with clipboard, or spiral-bound notebook, at the restaurant/bar/beach/hotel unattended all over the world and have never once had anyone mess with it. Contrast this with a computer, about which you will need to worry every hour of every day.

Similarly, I would leave other valuables (e.g., jewelry) at home. Sure, take a camera, but realize that you may not return with it.

Q **Suppose there is a person within sight in a uniform with a rifle or machine gun, and I want to take photos of a bridge, or a building, or anything else. What do I do?**

A Prior to your trip, learn how to say "Is taking a photograph permitted?" in the language spoken at your destinations. Walk to the person with rifle or machine gun (preferably not startling them from behind) and ask if you can shoot photos. They will say yes, in which case you shoot photos, or no, in which case you put your camera away. In many low-income nations, the definition of what represents a possible target of terrorism or insurgency is on the inclusive side, and if you take photos of something that is deemed sensitive—military barracks, military maneuvers, a police station, and so on—you could, at a minimum, have your camera confiscated and its memory card destroyed. I've spoken with travelers who have spent several hours with military or police, explaining why they were interested in whichever subjects they were photographing.

THE OLD MAGAZINE SCAM AND OTHER PETTY CRIME

I was at a bus station in Guatemala when a kid selling magazines approached me. The magazines were in English; each was plastic shrink-wrapped. They were pricey—four dollars for a *Newsweek* or *Harper's*—but I was facing a six-hour bus ride with nothing to read. I bought a *Time* for four bucks, and the kid vanished. Later, on the bus, as I was reading my magazine, something struck me as odd. What's this about William Casey having said something—wasn't he dead? And what's this about the Soviet Union—didn't that dissolve? I checked the date. The magazine was eight years old. The clever kid had stuck the price sticker over the date.

As scams go, this one was innocuous. I ended up reading it cover to cover about three times. (Did you know that Cary Grant and Desi Arnaz died in the same week in 1986?) Actually, I can't even say the kid lied—he didn't *say* the magazine was the current issue. If I assumed as much, well, that was my doing.

Have I myself ever been the victim of crime in a low- or middle-income nation? Yes. Once. I won't say which country, as you might deduce that that country is more dangerous than others, which it isn't. It was at a crowded bus station. My wallet was in my front pants pocket. I felt my arms momentarily pinned, a flick in my pocket, and my wallet was gone. By the time I realized what had happened, all I saw was people milling about me, and I had no idea who had taken it.

That's all that has happened in more than thirty years of trips to Central America and South America, Asia, and Africa. I was only a little irked. It wasn't brilliant of me to keep a wallet in a pants pocket. And I wasn't hurt. It was a hassle to cancel my credit card (which was not used—I assume they grabbed the cash and tossed the rest)—but otherwise it was a minor incident, albeit a lesson for me. I no longer use a wallet when I travel—I keep my money and passport in a belt around my waist (under pants and shirttails) or in a hotel safe deposit box.

Q This hotel has safe deposit boxes. Can I trust them?

A No strategy is foolproof, but hotel safe deposit boxes have an excellent record around the world. Hotels have a vested interest in keeping you from complaining to local police. Your belongings are almost certainly more safe in a hotel safe deposit box than on your person or in your hotel room.

Q I heard that sometimes taxi drivers kidnap tourists.

A This is rare, but it does happen. One strategy to employ is to have your hotel call for the cab. This will probably jack up the fare a tad, but drivers in taxis phoned by your hotel are much less likely to do you harm, relative to drivers of taxis that you hail randomly from the sidewalk. And—you did not hear this from me—if you do not have a local hotel, step into the first nice hotel you see and ask the concierge to call one for you. Usually staff at large hotels do not check to see if you're staying there or not. (Obviously this ploy fails at smaller establishments.) At airports, avoid "informal" taxis; instead, go to the official taxi queue.

Illicit Drug Use

A full one-third of the 2,500 US citizens who are arrested abroad each year are arrested on drug charges. A number of countries, including the Bahamas, the Dominican Republic, Jamaica, Mexico, and the Philippines, have enacted stringent drug laws that impose mandatory jail sentences for those convicted of possessing even small amounts of marijuana or cocaine for personal use. The death penalty remains an option in several countries, including Malaysia, Pakistan, and Turkey, for those caught smuggling illicit drugs.

If you are thinking that you might defray vacation expenses or augment your income by bringing back heroin, cocaine, or other illicit substances from abroad, see the 1978 movie *Midnight Express* for a fair warning.

Q **What about terrorism?**

A Terrorism makes the news because it's rare. In 2013, for example, sixteen US citizens were killed abroad by terrorism: thirteen in Afghanistan, two in Algeria, one in Lebanon. American citizens make over sixty million trips with at least one night outside the US each year. Your risk of dying of terrorism is infinitesimal and can be reduced further still by avoiding regions known to be tumultuous.

13

Jet Health

The Bottom Line

It is a paradoxical reality: In order to reach some remote, rural, and tranquil land, we must almost always first immerse ourselves in the cramped and noisy environment of the modern jet. We are grateful for these tin tubes of whoosh—without them we would spend most of our vacation traveling to and returning from our destinations—yet jets make us uncomfortable and crabby. Most of us do not hope for a good jet experience; we hope only to avoid Jet Godawfulness (delays, cancellations, hollering kid in close proximity for many hours).

A good strategy by which to feel minimally frazzled when you fly is to treat the entire experience like an endurance athletic event: wear comfortable clothes, drink a lot of water, avoid alcoholic beverages, sleep when you can.

Jet Lag

Most of us know jet lag. You fly west or east, the sun sets at the wrong time, you feel out of sorts for a few days, then you synch to the local day–night cycle only to repeat the pattern when you fly home. Symptoms include nighttime insomnia, daytime sleepiness, irritability, and inability to concentrate. It isn't debilitating, but it's a nuisance.

Our internal clock has a natural tendency to want to make our days a tad longer than twenty-four hours, and most people find that westward travel, which gives us a prolonged day, is easier than eastward travel, which shortens our day.

TO RESET YOUR INTERNAL CLOCK WITH BRIGHT LIGHT

- *For eastward travel:* While still in your locale of departure, get up earlier, and go to bed earlier, for two to three days prior to your trip. Expose yourself to bright light in the morning at your destination.
- *For westward travel:* While still in your locale of departure, go to bed later, and get up later, for two to three days prior to your trip. Expose yourself to bright light in the afternoon at your destination.

In fact, these measures are a pain and almost no one does this. When you travel through many time zones, it can take up to two weeks for your circadian clock to reset to the local light–dark cycle.

Very few studies have been done on the efficacy of the various measures intended to minimize jet lag; none has been done that compares the different measures to each other.

There also isn't much research on the well-being of jet passengers. In July 2007 the *New England Journal of Medicine* published a study in which five hundred healthy volunteers were placed in mock jets that were pressurized to the equivalent of various altitudes. Those exposed to the equivalent of 7,000 to 8,000 feet (2,130–2,440 meters) of altitude had more discomfort—backaches, headaches, shortness of breath, lightheadedness, and decreased coordination—than did those at the equivalent of lower altitudes; these differences became apparent after three to nine hours of simulated flight. This finding prompted Boeing to recommend that cabin air pressure in its 787 jets be set at the equivalent of 6,000 feet (1,830 meters), instead of the more usual 8,000 feet (2,440 meters).

176 ACTIVITIES AND ENVIRONS

Jet Health Q&A

Q **Jets make me uptight. I hate to fly. What should I do?**
A One option is to take zolpidem (Ambien) an hour prior to flights. It makes you tired, not comatose. If you take it, don't drive and stay away from alcoholic beverages. An advantage is that it has not been shown to affect your performance—mental or physical— the next day. This is opposed to diazepam (Valium), which can linger in you for several days. It also can be taken to help you to sleep on a jet.

Zolpidem (Ambien) is dispensed by prescription only. If flying makes you anxious, I think it's fully legit to ask your pre-travel provider to give you a prescription for a few tablets prior to your trip. The usual dose is 5 mg to 10 mg in men, 5 mg in women, 5 mg in the elderly.

As a rule, I don't like drugs in the benzodiazepine category (alprazolam [Xanax], diazepam [Valium])—they are, potentially, highly habit forming.

Q **I've heard great things about melatonin reducing or eliminating jet lag. Should I just take that to reset my clock?**
A This is controversial. On one hand, I've heard a number of reports from people who feel it reduces jet lag symptoms. (It isn't known if this is due to melatonin's effect as a soporific or as a hormone.) On the other hand, it's a hormone that has a number of influences on your body, and—here's why I come down on the "nay" side—studies are lacking. No one has taken a large group of international travelers and given them a standard dose and monitored them for efficacy and side effects. I do not recommend this hormone. I do not think it's been proven effective, and I do not think it's been proven to be safe. Given that we're talking about a condition that resolves after a few days without treatment, I'd vote for no drug at all. At some

point someone may do a randomized, placebo-controlled clinical trial and show that melatonin is great stuff. As of now, the jury's still out. Additionally, in the US melatonin tends to be sold at health food stores and is not regulated by the FDA; the result of this is that concentrations vary among different preparations, and, unlike drugs that the FDA regulates, potency may vary significantly among lots. In any case, children and pregnant women should avoid melatonin.

Some medical researchers distinguish between jet fatigue and jet lag. The former is characterized by general fatigue that resolves after a single night's sleep, and the latter is characterized by poor sleep that lasts for several days (about two-thirds as many days as time zones crossed for eastward travel; about half as many days as time zones crossed for westward travel).

Q I hate jet lag. Isn't there anything I can do to avoid it altogether?

A Sure. Instead of flying east or west, fly north or south. When you fly north or south there is no time change, hence no jet lag. Flights from Vancouver, British Columbia, to the Mexican state of Baja California, or New York to Lima, or London to Ghana, all occur in a single time zone.

Q What about blood clots? I read that jet passengers can get blood clots and die.

A Blood clots—usually originating in the legs, then traveling to the lungs, where they can be life threatening—are more common in jet passengers who fly for more than six hours, particularly in those who have preexisting risks for forming blood clots (obesity, history of previous blood clot, recent surgery, use of certain medications including birth control pills, and hormone replacement therapy). There is evidence that wearing pressure stockings (tight elastic stockings, such as TED hose and Jobst stockings with recommended pressures of 20–30 mmHg) reduces the risk of developing blood clots. Additionally, although no study has shown that these measures are of benefit, I think it's reasonable to keep well hydrated and walk frequently in an attempt to reduce risk.

A downside to taking a sedative such as Ambien is that you'll walk less—which could potentially increase the risk of blood clots.

Q **Should I take aspirin to reduce risk of blood clots?**
A Although intuitively this may make sense, it isn't recommended. (Studies showing safety and benefit have not been performed.)

Q **Is the air on jets super dry and filled with germs?**
A International travelers come down with the common cold and influenza more often than do folks who stay at home, so someone's coughing on them somewhere. Actually, jet cabin air is sucked through fine filters that should trap most germs.

Yes, jet air is very dry, which bothers some people. Keeping well hydrated, and putting saline drops into your eyes regularly, can help to alleviate symptoms brought on by this desert-like air.

Q **I have a head cold. Should I fly?**
A Although the odds of something bad (e.g., a ruptured eardrum) occurring when you fly with a head cold are minuscule, many people develop bothersome ear and/or sinus pain. The odds of this happening can be reduced by pre-flight decongestants, either by mouth (Actifed, Sudafed, Contac, others) or intra-nasally (Afrin). *Note:* Afrin should not be used for longer than three days due to the risk of rebound symptoms when it's stopped. Use Afrin as directed on the label the night before flying and the day of the flight. Most eustachian tube issues occur while descending in the plane, so chewing gum or sucking on a

hard candy as well as frequent swallowing during descent can help "pop" your ears and open up your eustachian tubes.

Because security rules change regarding what is allowable to carry on, travelers should always check the Transportation Security Administration's website at www.tsa.gov before traveling.

Q **I'm worried that the wings are going to fall off the jet and I'll plunge to my death.**

A Modern passenger jets are phenomenally safe. As has been said—it's a cliché but it's true—the most dangerous part of travel by air is the ride in the car to the airport.

In 2015, airlines carried 3.6 billion passengers on 29 million flights. There were sixteen fatal accidents, killing 560 people, meaning that your risk of dying on a passenger jet in 2015 was less than one in six million. Compare that to fifty years ago, when 87 crashes caused 1,597 deaths—and airlines carried only 5% of today's number of flights; 2016 was safer still; 2017, with 10 fatal commercial passenger and cargo air crashes that killed 44 people, safer still. In 2017, 80 million passengers flew for every commercial aviation death. Conclusion: Modern commercial aviation is extraordinarily safe.

Airlines based in high-income nations are safer than airlines based in low-income nations. But not everyone is comforted by statistics.

Q **I'm prone to motion sickness. Do drugs help?**

A Given sufficiently vigorous jostling and rocking, everyone is susceptible to motion sickness. Its symptoms are well known: cold sweats, nausea, vomiting.

If you plan to travel by boat and you're prone to motion sickness, you might consider a drug to help you to keep your lunch down. My favorite is "the patch": Transderm-scop (scopolamine), which is dispensed by prescription only. You put a small patch behind an ear; it lasts for three days, at which point you put a new one on if you're still at risk for motion sickness. The possible side effects include dry mouth and blurry vision.

Other prescription medications for motion sickness include promethazine (Phenergan) and prochlorperazine (former brand name: Compazine). These come as both tablets and rectal suppositories. A drawback of the tablets is that, potentially, you can vomit them up; they need to stay down for thirty to sixty minutes to be effective.

Q **What about those acupressure bracelets for motion sickness?**

A In clinical trials, bracelets do about as well at preventing motion sickness as do placebos—that is, not very well.

Q **What about over-the-counter drugs?**

A Several over-the-counter drugs have been shown to give some benefit to some people; options include diphenhydramine (Benadryl), dimenhydrinate (Dramamine), and meclizine (Antivert).

Hiking and High Altitude

The Bottom Line

- Hikers should carry the Ten Essentials.
- Acute mountain sickness (AMS) is common in travelers who ascend higher than 8,000 feet (2,440 meters); symptoms include headache, nausea, and a generally pissy mood.
- High-altitude cerebral edema (HACE) and high-altitude pulmonary edema (HAPE) are life-threatening conditions, the former causing confusion and clumsiness followed by coma, the latter causing a productive cough associated with decreased exercise tolerance and shortness of breath at rest.
- AMS generally resolves after a couple of days at altitude. The mainstay of treatment for HACE and HAPE is descent.

Hiking

To many travelers, the quintessential travel experience is to hoist a backpack and hike into terrain not accessible by car. Boy Scouts and Girl Scouts are taught the Ten Essentials they should carry for any outdoor activity (hiking, camping):

1. *Water.* This is probably the most important item on this list. If there is potentially potable water on your planned route, consider adding something lightweight with which to sterilize it (e.g., iodine tablets, filter, SteriPEN).
2. *Food.* High-calorie and lightweight (e.g., trail mix) is better than heavy (e.g., can of beans, watermelon).
3. *Matches and/or a fire starter.* One affordable brand of fire starter is Hot Spark Fire Starter, available from the Boy Scouts at www.scoutstuff.org. (*Note:* Mountain climbers should know where fires are and are not permitted on their planned route.)
4. *Pocket knife*
5. *First aid kit.* Adhesive bandages, tape, sterile gauze, moleskin (for blisters), soap, antiseptic, scissors. More extensive supplies are needed for more remote travel.
6. *Extra clothing.* Think layers.
7. *Sun protection.* Sunblock, lip block, sunglasses, wide-brimmed hat.
8. *Rain gear*
9. *Trail maps and compass*
10. *Flashlight or headlamp and extra batteries*
Optional: Consider adding a whistle and a cell phone.

Tell someone reliable (1) where you're going, (2) when you plan to return, and (3) when, should you not return on schedule, said reliable person should notify authorities and instigate a search.

Don't hike alone. Imitate scuba divers: Always travel with a buddy. Remember that guy who was hiking alone in a remote desert canyon in eastern Utah when a boulder trapped his hand? After a five-day wait, he performed an amputation at the forearm to escape. Had he been hiking with a buddy, that buddy could have trotted back for help.

Training is essential. A planned hike can be somewhat more strenuous than previous hikes but should not be markedly so. Particularly as we age we do better with gradual increases in activity, as opposed to attempting something prolonged and difficult with little or no training. Leapfrogging several levels of training is a good strategy by which to develop an overuse injury.

Treat your feet particularly well. Do not plan to hike in a brand-new pair of boots. Walk around in them for a few weeks first to make sure they're comfy.

Often the two-sock method will reduce risk of blisters. Wear a thin pair of polypro socks adjacent to skin, then a second pair of something thicker.

Pack a cheap and lightweight sheet of moleskin or some other blister adhesive strip in case of blisters.

When it comes to socks, wool is wise, cotton less so. Wool socks have advantages:

Wool is a better insulator than cotton.
Wool, unlike cotton, is insulating even when wet.
Wool can absorb a high amount of moisture, relative to cotton, before it feels wet.
Wool dries faster than cotton.
Wool is relatively odor resistant.

Good brand names of wool socks include SmartWool, Wigwam, and Thorlos.

Minimize your jewelry while hiking. Monkeys and birds can be attracted to shiny things, such as necklaces, bracelets, and earrings. You do not want monkeys or birds pulling your jewelry off.

Animal Attacks

Don't approach, pet, or feed wild animals. Whether or not it's permitted, it's a bad idea. Animal bites are not rare in travelers. A study performed at the international airport in Bangkok found that the rate of animal bites in travelers was a little over 1% per month of time abroad. Attacks by domestic animals are more common than attacks by animals in the wild; dogs are the most common animals to bite travelers. In addition to the physical injury of the bite, dogs can transmit rabies, a lethal viral infection. A dog's behavior is not a safe indicator as to whether or not it's rabid. ("Dumb" rabies, causing progressive paralysis, is more common in dogs than is "furious" rabies, in which the dog is highly excitable and chews on everything.)

The second most common animals to bite travelers are monkeys. Monkeys do not know that we are descended from a common primate ancestor and are hence genetic cousins (or they know but don't care). I have spoken with more than one traveler who has attempted to get a good photo of feeding a monkey, or a monkey on someone's lap or shoulder, only to receive (or sometimes photograph) a nasty bite. In addition to rabies, macaque monkeys often carry and can transmit herpes B, which can cause a lethal encephalitis (inflammation of the lining of the brain) in humans. Since 1932, there have been only fifty documented cases of herpes B in humans, but twenty-one of these were fatal. As many as 30% of feral rhesus macaque monkeys in Florida in state parks and elsewhere carry herpes B.

Virtually all wild animals, from squirrels to sea lions, can and will bite you if you attempt to cozy up too close. If you are bit or scratched by a wild animal, wash the bite site with soap and water, and seek immediate medical care, even if you have received the pre-exposure rabies series (see chapter 2). Specific antiviral prophylactic medication may be advised after a macaque monkey bite. Regarding snake bites, see chapter 18.

In bear country, keep food out of your tent and use the bear-resistant food containers if provided by a park; otherwise use a portable bear-resistant container or hang your food from a tree such that bears can't reach it. The US National Park Service has helpful info on storing food and other things that bears might eat at https://www.nps.gov/subjects/bears/storingfood.htm.

For a particularly vivid lesson on the downside of getting too close to wild animals, see Werner Herzog's 2005 film *Grizzly Man*. It tells the tale of American Timothy Treadwell, who lived amongst grizzly bears in Alaska's Katmai National Park during summers. At the end of his thirteenth summer in the park a bear ate both him and his girlfriend, Amie Huguenard.

Hiking Q&A

Q **I've sprained my ankle in the past. How do I avoid recurrent ankle sprains?**
A Home-based proprioceptive training programs have been shown to reduce risk, as does wearing an ankle brace. Boots may provide stability as well.

Q **What about electrolytes? Should I drink electrolyte-rich drinks and/or take electrolyte tablets such as Nuun?**
A No. Food and water are better. If you're eating three meals a day, you don't need additional electrolytes.

Q **Any issues with low-humidity hikes?**
A Some regions, including deserts and alpine mountains, can have very low humidity, which can predispose visitors to nosebleeds (epistaxis). This can be prevented by nasal saline gel spray a few times per day, as well as applying nasal gel to the inner nostrils and nasal septum—the cartilage wall between the nostrils.

Altitude Illness

There are three illnesses of high altitude—above 8,000 feet (2,440 meters)—that you should be aware of. One is common and minor (acute mountain sickness); the other two are rare and life threatening (high-altitude cerebral edema and high-altitude pulmonary edema).

ACUTE MOUNTAIN SICKNESS (AMS)

Acclimatization is the process by which your body becomes adapted to breathing the thin air of high altitude. You breathe faster and deeper, your heart beats more quickly, your body produces more red blood cells to carry oxygen from your lungs to the rest of your body. All this takes several days to kick in, which is why many new arrivals to altitude experience the symptoms of acute mountain sickness. AMS is the most common altitude-related ailment of those at high altitude. It occurs in about a quarter of Colorado resort skiers and over half of those who climb Mount Rainier (14,410 feet [4,390 meters]) in Washington State. It is more common in those who ascend quickly, as well as in those who have had it before. Men are a bit more prone to this than are women. Interestingly, although being physically fit improves your comfort and performance at altitude, it does not lessen your odds of AMS.

Many people who ascend quickly, or fly from sea level to high altitude, find themselves experiencing headache, nausea, and general malaise; it is often likened to a hangover. This usually commences between a few hours to a few days after arrival at altitude; it goes away after a few days if you remain at altitude, or after return to low altitude. It does not usually lead to anything serious, but it's unpleasant and can keep you in bed. Risk is reduced by ascending slowly (no more than 1,500 feet [460 meters]/day), taking a rest day at 10,000 feet (3,050 meters) and every three to four days thereafter, and/or by taking acetazolamide (see below).

HIGH-ALTITUDE CEREBRAL EDEMA (HACE)

A small number of people with AMS will progress to HACE. HACE usually develops a few days after the onset of AMS. It is rare below 10,000 feet (3,050 meters). As with AMS and HAPE, rapid ascent is a risk factor. Signs and symptoms include an unsteady gait, faulty judgment, bizarre behavior, hallucinations, severe headache, and lethargy, which can progress to coma and death. HACE and HAPE can occur simultaneously.

HIGH-ALTITUDE PULMONARY EDEMA (HAPE)

As many as 1% to 2% of people who travel above 12,000 feet (3,660 meters) develop HAPE. Sometimes it follows AMS, or it can occur without prior warning. HAPE occurs most commonly two to five days after ascent to altitude. The cardinal sign of HAPE is decreased exercise performance: You can't keep up with others (whereas formerly you could), you need more breaks than others, and you don't recover on breaks.

Risk factors for HAPE include rapid ascent, marked exertion on arrival, and having had HAPE in the past. You can greatly reduce your odds of all three of the above by ascending gradually. If you ascend by only 1,500 feet (460 meters) per day, these illnesses are markedly less likely. But most of us are only able to get away for a few days and tend to ascend with alacrity. For example, the great majority of people who want to see Machu Picchu, the Inca site in the Peruvian Andes, fly from Lima, at sea level, to Cuzco, at 11,152 feet (3,400 meters). Similarly most of those who summit on Mount Rainier climb the first day from Paradise, at 5,400 feet (1,650 meters), to Camp Muir, at 10,080 feet (3,070 meters), then quickly summit at 14,410 feet (4,390 meters) the following morning—hence the high rate of AMS in those who climb Mount Rainier.

Recall that who takes care of whom is dictated by circumstance. Suppose you're climbing a mountain with a doctor who gets a bad headache and then begins to act weird (or weirder than usual). You've just been promoted. Now *you're* the doctor. Your plan should be to descend with the doctor, who may very well have HACE (high-altitude cerebral edema), regardless of what that doctor wants to do.

Travelers should suspect significant altitude illness in *themselves* if they experience any of the following:

- A headache and hungover feeling
- Shortness of breath and a respiratory rate of more than twenty breaths/minute while at rest
- Markedly decreased appetite
- Vomiting
- Clumsiness
- Unusual fatigue while walking

Travelers should suspect significant altitude illness in their *companions* who are:

- Skipping meals
- Not friendly, although they were friendly in the past
- Stumbling or otherwise newly klutzy
- Having difficulty doing a straightforward activity
- Arriving last at the daily destination and being the most fatigued
- Short of breath at rest
- Having hallucinations or confusion

Based on Stephen A. Bezruchka, "Altitude Illness," in E. C. Jong and R. McMullen, eds., *The Travel and Tropical Medicine Manual*, 3rd ed. (Philadelphia: Saunders/Elsevier, 2003).

TREATMENT OF ACUTE MOUNTAIN SICKNESS

Mild AMS can be treated by conservative measures: staying at the same altitude until symptoms resolve (usually one to two days), followed by cautious ascent. Symptoms can be reduced by nonnarcotic analgesics (acetaminophen [Tylenol] or ibuprofen [Advil, Motrin]), relative rest, and advancing activities as tolerated. Acetazolamide (Diamox) 250 mg, twice a day, also usually helps.

Note: The treatment dose for AMS, acetazolamide 250 mg twice a day, is double the prevention dose of 125 mg twice a day. Generally, only two or three days of this are needed; after a few days at altitude your body's natural acclimatization mechanisms begin to kick in. If AMS seems severe, or doesn't resolve after two to three days, descend.

TREATMENT OF HAPE AND HACE

To treat HAPE or HACE, it is most important to descend. Oxygen, if available, will help, as will the use of a hyperbaric bag (a portable bag that encloses the patient; the bag is then inflated such that the pressure is equivalent to that at a lower altitude). One type of hyperbaric bag is the Gamow bag. Dexamethasone for HACE and nifedipine (Procardia) for HAPE (see more info in the High-Altitude Pharmacology section that follows) are also of benefit but should be used only in conjunction with descent.

TIPS FOR PREVENTING ALTITUDE ILLNESS

If you want to prevent AMS, HAPE, and HACE, the best thing you can do is ascend slowly. There is no correct rate of ascent; everyone responds differently to altitude. During ascent, you should monitor yourself and your companions for signs and symptoms of altitude illness. Additionally:

- Climb high but sleep low. The altitude at which you sleep should rise gradually. A conservative rate of ascent would be to take two days to get to 10,000 feet (3,050 meters), then to raise the altitude at which you sleep by no more than 1,000 feet (305 meters) per night.
- If you have a headache, never ascend to sleep.
- Anyone who is clumsy, confused, or short of breath at rest needs to descend to below the altitude at which the symptoms began. A good test for clumsiness is the "heel–toe" walk

in which you walk a straight line, touching your heel to the toe of your other foot. (This is what the police make you do to prove your sobriety.)

- Carry drugs for high-altitude illness (see the High-Altitude Pharmacology section).
- Avoid sedatives, tranquilizers, and narcotic analgesics. These drugs may blunt your body's natural inclination to breathe deeply while at high altitude. Examples include alcoholic beverages, diazepam (Valium), alprazolam (Xanax), and codeine and other opiates.
- Drink a lot of fluids. Fluids don't prevent AMS, but adequate fluids prevent dehydration, which can feel similar.
- Avoid strenuous overexertion while at altitude.
- Wear appropriate clothing—that is, keep warm. Hypothermia worsens altitude illness. The average temperature drop as you ascend is 3.5°F per 1,000 feet (0.65°C/100 meters).
- Do not assist someone in climbing higher. If someone is having trouble climbing, it may be due to altitude illness. Carrying or pulling someone to a higher altitude may be the worst thing you could do. And don't leave someone alone in a remote or high-altitude area—they may worsen and require assistance.

Based on Stephen A. Bezruchka, "Altitude Illness," in E. C. Jong and R. McMullen, eds., *The Travel and Tropical Medicine Manual*, 3rd ed. (Philadelphia: Saunders/Elsevier, 2003).

High-Altitude Pharmacology

ACETAZOLAMIDE

Acetazolamide is a weak diuretic—that is, it makes you urinate a little more. Although its primary role is to treat glaucoma, a condition in which the pressure inside the eye is elevated, it is also used to lessen the risk of AMS.

People in the moderate- and high-risk categories (see the Risk Categories for Acute Mountain Sickness feature) should consider taking acetazolamide preventatively. In recent years, the recommended dose for this purpose has decreased; the current advised dose is 125 mg, twice per day, for a minimum of three days, beginning one day prior to ascent. It can be stopped a couple of days after your top altitude is reached. Although it's only a weak diuretic at this dose, I suggest you take the doses early in the day (say 8:00 a.m. and 2:00 p.m.); this appears not to impact the benefit, while minimizing the diuretic side effect at night, when it's least convenient.

Risk Categories for Acute Mountain Sickness

RISK CATEGORY	DESCRIPTION
Low	Individuals with no prior history of altitude illness and ascending to ≤ 9,200 feet (2,800 meters)
	Individuals taking ≥ 2 days to arrive at 8,200–9,800 feet (2,500–3,000 meters) with subsequent increases in sleeping elevation < 1,640 feet (500 meters)/day and an extra day for acclimatization every 3,280 feet (1,000 meters)
Moderate	Individuals with prior history of AMS and ascending to 8,200–9,200 feet (2,500–2,800 meters) in 1 day
	No history of AMS and ascending to > 9,200 feet (2,800 meters) in 1 day
	All individuals ascending > 1,640 feet (500 meters)/day (increase in sleeping elevation) at altitudes above 9,800 feet (3,000 meters) but with an extra day for acclimatization every 3,280 feet (1,000 meters)

High	Individuals with a history of AMS and ascending to > 9,200 feet (2,800 meters) in 1 day
	All individuals with a prior history of HACE
	All individuals ascending to > 11,500 feet (3,500) meters in 1 day
	All individuals ascending > 1,640 feet (500 meters)/day (increase in sleeping elevation) above > 9,800 feet (3,000 meters) without extra days for acclimatization
	Very rapid ascents (e.g., < 7-day ascents of Mount Kilimanjaro)

Source: A. M. Luks, S. E. McIntosh, C. K. Grissom, P. S. Auerbach, G. W. Rodway, R. B. Schoene, K. Zafren, and P. H. Hackett. "Wilderness Medical Society Practice Guidelines for the Prevention and Treatment of Acute Altitude Illness: 2014 Update," *Wilderness and Environmental Medicine,* vol. 25, number 4.

Additionally, acetazolamide can be used to treat AMS. It is entirely reasonable to take nothing preventatively, determine whether or not you develop AMS, then take acetazolamide if you do. The dose and schedule for treatment is 250 mg twice per day for a minimum of three days. If you stop the medication at altitude and symptoms reoccur, it is fine to take it for a few more days.

If you ascend slowly (no more than 1,500 feet [460 meters] per day), there is usually no need to take acetazolamide.

Another use for acetazolamide is to treat the poor sleep that develops at high altitude. Poor sleep is almost universal at high altitude; it usually improves after three or four nights at a given altitude. Acetazolamide 125 mg at bedtime significantly improves the quality of sleep for those experiencing restless nights at high altitude.

There is one innocuous, albeit weird, side effect of acetazolamide. While you're taking it, you can't tell the difference between carbonated and not carbonated drinks. This is unlikely to affect your life unless you're a taster at a pop factory, but still, it's odd; I don't know of another drug with this side effect. In fact, while you're taking it, try drinking a carbonated pop or a beer. It'll taste off—not horrendous, just not right. The side effect quickly vanishes after you finish the drug. Another side effect of acetazolamide for some is tingling in the hands and feet and around the mouth; this quickly resolves after reducing the dose or stopping the medication.

Acetazolamide can occasionally make you drowsy or sun sensitive. Additional potential side effects include dizziness, lightheadedness, blurred vision, loss of appetite, and nausea. It is not approved for use during pregnancy. Acetazolamide is available in generic form and hence is inexpensive.

DEXAMETHASONE

Dexamethasone, a steroid, prevents and treats AMS and HACE; it also reduces risk of HAPE. If you can't tolerate acetazolamide, taking dexamethasone to prevent AMS is an option. However, if dexamethasone is stopped at high altitude, rebound symptoms may occur. Taking dexamethasone to prevent altitude illness is not routinely recommended.

Unlike acetazolamide, steroids including dexamethasone have a plethora of side effects. You can become euphoric and make unwise decisions (such as continuing to climb at dusk). Your mood can crash when you stop taking it. It sends your blood glucose up. Long-term users see even more problems.

STEROID RECAP

- If you do suffer signs and/or symptoms of severe AMS or HACE and take dexamethasone or another steroid, recall that the most important part of treatment is descent.
- The usual dexamethasone dose is 4 mg every six hours; this needs to be tapered down when discontinued if it is taken more than three weeks.

NIFEDIPINE

Nifedipine can be used to either prevent or treat HAPE. It is usually recommended only for people who have had HAPE in the past. The dose for prevention or treatment of HAPE is 30 mg extended release every twelve hours; for prevention start twenty-four hours before ascent.

SILDENAFIL, TADALAFIL

Either sildenafil (Viagra) or tadalafil (Cialis) are alternate drugs that can be taken to prevent or treat HAPE. The sildenafil dose is 50 mg every eight hours; the tadalafil dose is 10 mg every twelve hours.

Climbing Gear

Air invariably gets cooler as you ascend. That, combined with the potential for worsening weather, means you should always pack multiple layers of cold-weather gear when you climb.

Look at the gear of the other climbers. If everyone else is carrying ice axes and wearing crampons and quintuple-thick parkas and you're in a tank top and tennis shoes, rethink your equipment.

High-Altitude Medicine Q&A

Q I didn't get altitude illness the last time I climbed, so I won't get it in the future, right?

A Prior performance is a good, but not perfect, predictor. If you did well on a prior hike and repeat it—identical altitude, identical rate of ascent—you'll probably do okay. If you climb a little faster, all bets are off.

Q So the biggest threats to my health as I climb are cerebral and pulmonary edema?

A No. The most common cause of death of mountaineers is falls. The best way to ensure your safety is to know what you're doing and to avoid attempting to climb a mountain that requires skills beyond your level. Rope up when you need to, take appropriate gear, including ice ax and crampons, and—as readers of Jon Krakauer's *Into Thin Air* know—adhere to your turn-back time, even if you haven't summited. It is better to descend and climb another day than to attain a summit only to leave your carcass on the mountain.

Q If I develop AMS and do nothing, will it go away?

A Yes, usually in one to two days.

Q How can I tell AMS from HACE?

A Headache, possibly accompanied by nausea but clearheaded and not clumsy = AMS. Confusion and/or clumsiness (e.g., unsteady gait) = HACE.

Q Can I acclimatize to any altitude?

A No, only to about 18,000 feet (5,500 meters). There are no permanent human habitations above 18,000 feet.

Q As I climb, is there anything other than thin air I need to contend with?

A Yes, increased ultraviolet (UV) radiation. UV radiation increases by 4% for every 1,000 feet (305 meters) of altitude gain, increasing your risk of sunburn. Cover up, and use high-SPF sun block on exposed skin.

Q Anything else?

A Decreased humidity, which, in combination with hyperventilation, can result in dehydration, is a potential issue. Drinking adequate fluids is key.

Q Can I use herbal supplements to prevent or treat altitude illness?

A There is no evidence that coca tea, garlic, ginkgo biloba, or vitamin E are of benefit. *Note:* Drinking even a single cup of coca tea will give you a positive result for cocaine metabolites for several days on routine drug toxicology screening.

15

Swimming and Diving

The Bottom Line

To breathe underwater and bond with our fish forebears (the "finny tribes" per Melville) is fundamentally cool. However, scuba diving presents significant risks over snorkeling. If, for example, you take a breath at depth, then ascend while holding your breath, you will be, in the parlance of my military friends, DRT: dead right there.

Two categories of medical problems that stem from diving are barotrauma, which is caused by expansion or compression of gas within gas-filled body compartments, and decompression illness, which is caused by nitrogen bubbles formed after breathing air under increased pressure.

Concerning animals and plants you will see underwater, pretend you're in a really expensive store: Look, but don't touch.

Membership in one or more diving professional organizations can help you keep up to date regarding diving health—see the Resources for International Travelers section at the end of this guide.

Swimming Safety

Drowning is the second-most common cause of non-elderly travelers' deaths, after road traffic injuries. Following these tips will reduce risk:

- Swim in designated areas supervised by lifeguards.
- Swim with a buddy.
- Know how to swim. If you don't know how to swim, enroll in a class prior to your trip.
- Travel with a cell phone; know how to call the local emergency number.
- Beware of rip currents (also known as riptides and undertow). Rip currents are powerful currents of water flowing away from shore. They can occur at any beach with breaking waves. If caught in a rip current, don't fight it, but swim out of it, parallel to shore.
- Don't swim after drinking alcoholic beverages.

Adapted from *American Red Cross: Swimming Safety Tips*, available at www.redcross.org/get-help/how-to-prepare-for-emergencies /types-of-emergencies/water-safety/swim-safety.

Scuba Diving

Scuba diving is tremendous fun, but it is a relatively high-risk sport. Even within the US, 3 to 9 divers per 100,000 die each year. Those over age 45 should have a physical examination, and a stress EKG (i.e., a treadmill test) prior to their first dive. Although sport diving has no formal age restriction, most certification programs begin at age 12. A high level of emotional maturity is essential to participate in this sport.

Training, ideally, involves several weeks of classroom presentations, pool training, and open-water diving. Many authorities believe that weekend courses, often offered at tourist resorts, are inadequate.

Also—this may sound simplistic, but I'll emphasize it nonetheless: You should know how to swim. The most common cause of death of scuba divers is not barotrauma or decompression illness—it is drowning, which accounts for 60% of diving deaths. To be sure, not all drowning deaths are due to an inability to swim, but nonetheless it is undeniably improvident to scuba unless you are a good swimmer. (See the Contraindications to Scuba Diving feature for a full list of medical contraindications to scuba diving.)

If you don't scuba, you only snorkel, you can skip ahead to the Marine Hazards section.

CONTRAINDICATIONS TO SCUBA DIVING

Physicians talk about two types of contraindications: absolute and relative. Absolute contraindications are those that bar everyone with that condition from diving; people with the conditions listed as relative contraindications may be able to scuba dive after consultation with their physicians.

ABSOLUTE CONTRAINDICATIONS

- Seizure disorder (epilepsy). A history of febrile seizures as a child is not a contraindication. Consider obtaining a brain wave test (EEG) after head trauma.
- Myocardial infarction (heart attack) within the previous year, symptomatic coronary artery disease (angina), congestive heart failure, atrial septal defect, history of stroke, uncontrolled hypertension.
- Uncontrolled depression, schizophrenia, anxiety or panic disorders, history of psychosis or suicide attempt; children with uncontrolled hyperactivity disorder.
- Sickle cell disease (homozygous).
- Unexplained fainting.
- Dizziness.
- Inability to equalize middle ear pressures (painlessly "pop" your ears).
- Chronic lung disease such as bullous emphysema; previous episode of POPS (pulmonary overpressurization syndrome); history of spontaneous pneumothorax.

- Tympanic membrane (ear drum) perforation, unless healed or surgically repaired.
- Pregnancy.

RELATIVE CONTRAINDICATIONS

- Asthma. This is somewhat controversial. You should discuss your asthma with your healthcare provider prior to diving; that provider may obtain pulmonary function tests (PFTs) prior to your diving.
- Diabetes. Those with poor control and/or hypoglycemic episodes should not dive.
- Mitral valve prolapse.
- Migraine headaches. Those with an active headache should not dive.
- Limited vision. Wearing contact lenses is safe; divers who have had radial keratotomy should wait two to five months after the procedure before diving. (Previously repaired retinal detachment and controlled glaucoma are not contraindications.)
- Patients with recent surgery are usually okay to dive after they are without symptoms but should be cleared by their surgeons prior to diving.
- Inguinal or abdominal hernias should be repaired prior to diving.
- Respiratory infections, either upper (e.g., bronchitis) or lower (e.g., pneumonia) are temporary contraindications.
- Sickle cell disease (heterozygous).

Adapted from A. Spira, "Diving and Marine Medicine," in J. Keystone, P. Kozarsky, D. O. Freedman, H. Nothdurft, & B. Connor, *Travel Medicine* (Edinburgh: Mosby, 2004).

Barotrauma

Barotrauma affects body areas filled with air or other gases. These include the middle ear (the air-containing space of the ear bordered on one side by the tympanic membrane), Eustachian tubes, sinuses, lungs, and gastrointestinal tract. Either descending, when the pressure of the water is greater than the pressure in these cavities, or ascending, when the pressure of water is less than that of these cavities, can cause symptoms.

The most common site of barotrauma is the middle ear. Pressure can be equalized only via the Eustachian tube, which goes between the throat and the middle ear. If the Eustachian tube is blocked by a head cold, allergies, or another cause, you won't be able to equalize the pressure in your middle ear, and pain, and possible rupture of your eardrum, will result.

Middle ear squeeze occurs during descent, usually in the first 33 feet (10 meters), when the Eustachian tube is blocked; the eardrum pushes in, causing pain. If the diver ignores initial pain and continues to descend, the eardrum may rupture, allowing cold water to rush into the middle ear, which can cause vertigo, nausea, and vomiting, which can be fatal while diving. If descending divers cannot equalize pressure between the throat and middle ears via patent (open, unblocked) Eustachian tubes (which will manifest as ear pain during descent), they must ascend to the depth at which equalization is possible, then slowly descend again.

Reverse squeeze occurs when a diver tries to ascend with a blocked Eustachian tube; the gas expands with ascent, pushing the eardrum outward and causing pain. One cause of this is the diver taking decongestants that wear off while diving. As with squeeze that occurs on descent, reverse squeeze can lead to pain, hemorrhage, and/or rupture of the eardrum.

The second most common site of barotraumas is the sinuses. Ordinarily, the ostia (little holes in the skull that allow mucus to drain from sinuses into the nasal cavity) are patent, such that air can travel freely between the nose and the sinuses. If these are blocked from allergies, a head cold, or other causes, the air in the sinuses is sealed off and tends to contract during descent and expand during ascent. When this happens, your head does not explode but it will occur to you that it might.

Upper respiratory infections, allergies, nasal polyps, overuse of nasal spray (vasoconstrictor sprays such as oxymetazoline [Afrin], not steroid sprays such as fluticasone propionate [Flonase]), tobacco use, and anatomic abnormalities such as a deviated septum may predispose individuals to sinus barotrauma.

Air in the gastrointestinal tract will expand as a diver ascends, stretching the intestines, which can be uncomfortable; belches and farts may ensue. This is more common in novice divers, who are more prone to swallowing air while underwater, and those who drink carbonated drinks or eat a large meal immediately pre-dive, which should be avoided.

Tooth squeeze (tooth pain) arises from small pockets of air in dental cavities, defective caps or crowns, temporary fillings, or gum infections. The air contracts as you descend and expands as you ascend, causing pain, and, in extreme cases, implosion of the tooth during descent or explosion during ascent. Divers should maintain excellent dental health and avoid diving with a temporary crown.

Mask squeeze is caused by insufficient air pressure in the mask during descent. This can lead to subconjunctival hemorrhages (bleeding in the lining over the whites of your eyes), and bruising around your eyes. Although this will make you look like you've been mugged, it isn't harmful and resolves in a few days. Prevention is accomplished by exhaling slightly into the mask during descent.

Pulmonary Over-Pressurization Syndrome

The appropriate acronym POPS (pulmonary over-pressurization syndrome), also known as burst lung, arises from gas expansion that exceeds the lungs' ability to expand. This causes rupture of tissue at the level of the alveoli, which are the tiny gas-filled sacs in your lungs where gases are exchanged with your blood. POPS consists of some combination of four components: arterial gas embolism (gas bubbles in the arteries), pneumomediastinum (air in the space in the chest between the lungs), pneumothorax (air between a lung and the lining of the lungs), and subcutaneous emphysema (air under skin).

In normal lungs, POPS is most often due to breath holding during ascent or shooting to the surface too quickly to allow you to exhale expanding gas. A number of illnesses and conditions predispose to POPS, including chronic obstructive pulmonary disease (COPD), specifically emphysema and chronic bronchitis; acute bronchitis; and asthma.

Arterial gas embolism is the most significant danger posed by POPS; it is second only to drowning as a cause of death of divers. When alveoli burst from expanding gas, bubbles of air move into the arteries, where they travel, then lodge in arterioles (small arteries) and/or capillaries (smaller blood vessels still). Usually this condition is noted within ten minutes of surfacing and is suggested by bloody froth at the mouth and/or chest pain. When these air emboli lodge in the brain, they can cause pretty much any neurological or psychiatric condition you can think of, including vertigo, headache, visual changes, sensory changes, confusion, personality changes, paralysis, seizures, stroke, and death.

If the air emboli lodge in the heart, they can cause a myocardial infarction (heart attack); if they lodge in the spinal cord, numbness or paralysis may result. If arterial gas embolism occurs while a diver is underwater, it is often fatal. It can occur in dives as shallow as 3 feet (1 meter) or after dives of only a few seconds.

Therapy consists of immediate recompression in a compression chamber; however, these are often not available outside of urban centers. Prior to their trip, divers should learn the whereabouts of the one nearest their dive site.

The Bends

As a diver breathes pressurized air, nitrogen is absorbed into body tissues; as a diver ascends, this gas comes out of solution. If a diver ascends too quickly, this gas forms bubbles in blood or body tissues, causing the bends, more formally known as decompression sickness (DCS). The bubbles tend to be in veins, not arteries. This does not occur in shallow water. Factors increasing the risk of bends, in addition to ascending too quickly, include diving for too long a duration or at a depth beyond no-decompression diving, dehydration, advanced age, obesity, previous injury, alcohol use, and cold. Bubbles can block blood vessels or cause uncontrolled clotting of blood (disseminated intravascular coagulation). A number of tables (e.g., the US Navy Guide Tables) provide guidelines for safe depth and dive duration to avoid the bends; however, sometimes a diver can follow these guidelines and develop the bends nonetheless.

If a diver plans a number of dives on a given day, doing the deepest dive first reduces risk of the bends.

Decompression sickness can manifest as a number of syndromes: pain syndromes, spinal cord syndrome, cerebral syndrome, peripheral nerve syndrome, and dysbaric osteonecrosis (bubbles in blood vessels in bone, causing death of bone tissue). As a general rule, the sooner the symptoms occur after a dive, the more severe they tend to be and the faster they tend to progress.

Decompression sickness (DCS) is divided into two categories of severity: DCS I, which consists of rash and/or muscle or joint pain only, and the more serious DCS II. The most common form of bends is pain in muscles and joints (DCS I). Shoulders, elbows, and arms are the most common site of pain. The presence of any neurological, cardiac, or pulmonary symptoms puts the diver into the category of DCS II. Symptoms of DCS II include altered or decreased skin sensation, weakness, inability to urinate, confusion, unsteadiness of gait, visual changes, and chest pain and cough ("the chokes").

The neurologic symptoms are most frequently due to spinal cord involvement; symptoms include lower back pain, abdominal pain, leg weakness, and altered skin sensation. Some symptoms may persist after recompression therapy.

DCS affecting the inner ear is termed *vestibular decompression sickness* ("the staggers"—divers utilize vivid terms for their ailments). This consists of dizziness, ringing in the ears, decreased hearing, and nausea. Any of these symptoms constitutes a medical emergency; immediate recompression in a compression chamber is necessary.

Travel in jets, which are usually pressurized to the equivalent of 6,000 to 8,000 feet (1,830 to 2,440 meters) of altitude, not sea level, can facilitate the occurrence of the bends; most authorities advise that divers not fly for at least twenty-four hours after diving.

Nitrogen Narcosis

Nitrogen narcosis, which Jacques Cousteau termed *rapture of the deep*, stems from nitrogen's propensity to act as a narcotic when under pressure. Basically, you get a little loopy when you dive below about 100 feet. Dive physicians jocularly refer to the Martini effect, or Martini's Law, which states that every 33 feet (10 meters) of descent below about 100 feet (30 meters) is equivalent, in terms of the narcotic effect of nitrogen, to drinking one martini. This effect is exacerbated by exercise, cold, fear, and, as you would expect, pre-dive alcoholic beverages. Divers who make repeated deep dives develop partial tolerance. Symptoms resolve after ascent.

Hypoxemia and Hyperoxemia

Either too little or too much oxygen (hypoxemia and hyperoxemia, respectively) presents a threat to divers. Breathing pure oxygen at depths over 33 feet (10 meters) can cause seizures, which can lead to aspiration of water or drowning. Short exposures of breathing pure oxygen under elevated pressure can cause any number of neurological symptoms, including abnormal vision, tinnitus (ringing in the ears), dizziness, and nausea.

Marine Hazards

Concerning animals and plants you will see underwater, as a general rule, it's not a good idea to reach out and touch stuff when you're diving. A surprising number of things you might encounter underwater—fish, coral, plants, and more—will bite, sting, or otherwise cause you pain.

Cnidaria (pronounced nye-DARE-ee-uh; the *c* is silent) is a phylum containing jellyfish, sea anemones, and corals; many members of this phylum are able to cause stings ranging from mild to deadly. Coral and anemones cause burning and itching; jellyfish can cause symptoms ranging from pain to shock and even death.

Jellyfish stings are more common when diving off a downwind shore and during jellyfish blooms, when jellyfish are present in large number. Many jellyfish stings are mild, causing only redness and pain, and can be treated without involving medical professionals. The area that was stung should be washed immediately with seawater; applying fresh water may cause further symptoms. Vinegar, which neutralizes stingers still on the skin, should then be applied (with exceptions noted below). Remaining stingers can be removed by applying shaving cream, or a paste of seawater and baking soda, or sea water and talcum powder to the skin, allowing it to dry, then scraping it off. Applying ice and skin creams such as calamine lotion reduces pain and itching.

Jellyfish causing severe symptoms include the box jellyfish, found in Pacific and Caribbean waters, and the Portuguese man o' war, also known as the bluebottle jellyfish, which has a distinctive purple bubble on its upper surface that serves as a sail; it is found on both the Atlantic and Pacific Coasts of North America, off Hawaii, and in the Gulf of Mexico. Other jellyfish causing severe symptoms include the sea nettle, a brown or red jellyfish that is common off the Atlantic shore of the US, and the lion's mane, the world's largest jellyfish, which can reach diameters of 8 feet (2.4 meters); it usually resides in the cooler, northern waters of the Pacific and Atlantic Oceans. A particularly deadly species of box jellyfish is the sea wasp (*Chironex fleckeri*), found in waters off northern Queensland, Australia, as well as New Guinea and the Philippines. Stings are extremely painful; severe (large area) stings can be fatal within as little as three minutes. More than sixty sea wasp–caused deaths in Australia have been recorded.

Vinegar is not of benefit for Pacific Portuguese man o' war, and it actually activates nematocysts (specialized cells containing barbed, threadlike tubes that sting) in the Atlantic Portuguese man o' war. It should not be applied to sea nettle stings.

After stings from box jellyfish, treatment with *Chironex* antivenom can be lifesaving; as a rule, however, this is available only in Australia. In the event that the heart of someone stung by a box jellyfish stops, CPR should be performed; the toxins from box jellyfish are heat labile (degrade in something as warm as a person), and favorable outcomes have occurred even after prolonged CPR.

Wearing women's nylon pantyhose over arms and legs will prevent jellyfish from stinging. In Australia you will not infrequently see lifeguards wearing pantyhose on all four limbs. It looks odd but is an easy way to prevent stings. Experts debate the mechanism of protection. Some jellyfish have very short stingers that can't penetrate the nylon mesh; the stingers of other jellyfish are triggered by contact with the surface of the skin and the nylon provides sufficient buffer such that skin is protected. Specially made stinger suits, also widely used in Australia, are fully protective.

Cuts and scrapes on coral frequently become infected due to a high bacterial count in the coral. Vigorous cleaning after the fact is helpful, but many people require antibiotics, either topical or oral, following abrasions or puncture wounds by coral.

Scorpionfishes, lionfishes (often sold at tropical fish stores), and stonefishes have venom gland–bearing fin rays. The good news is that they use these only for defense; they are not aggressors under ordinary conditions. However, if you handle one in an aquarium, or step on one in the ocean, they often sting, causing immediate and intense pain. Treatment consists of non-scalding hot water (up to 113°F/45°C), irrigation of the wound, removal of spine and sheath fragments, and seeing a medical professional. Wounds should not be sutured closed as this increases risk of infection. Those with deep wounds and all wounds to the hand or foot, which are at elevated risk of infection, should be treated with a preventative antibiotic.

Sea urchin spines are sharp and brittle; they often lodge deeply into skin and muscle and are difficult to remove. Many have venom in the spines, exposure to which causes anything from minor skin redness to extreme pain with nausea, vomiting, decreased blood pressure, fainting, and respiratory compromise. Immersion of the affected area into non-scalding hot water (up to 113°F/45°C) for thirty to ninety minutes offers significant initial relief from pain.

Some starfish are soft and squishy, some have big thorns, some are venomous. The crown-of-thorns starfish, *Acanthaster planci*, is particularly nasty. It is found around coral reefs of the Pacific and Indian Oceans, the Gulf of California, the Red Sea, and the Great Barrier Reef. Its spines, which can grow to 2.5 inches (6 centimeters), are covered with venom and can easily penetrate diving gloves. Pain, bleeding, and swelling occur after penetration of the skin by spines of the crown-of-thorns starfish; penetration by multiple spines can cause altered skin sensation, vomiting, and paralysis. Treatment is supportive: non-scalding hot water (as described above) and pain medications.

Some octopuses (the plural form *octopi* is no longer favored) are venomous. Bites with their parrot-shaped beaks are rarely severe, but bites of the greater blue-ringed octopus, *Hapalochlaena lunulata*, and the southern blue-ringed octopus (also known as the Australian spotted octopus), *Hapalochlaena maculosa*, can be life threatening. Found in coastal waters and tide pools around Australia, these small octopuses—8 inches (20 centimeters) with their tentacles extended— are not out to get you. Most bites occur when they are picked up or stepped on. When they bite, symptoms include nausea, vomiting, blurred vision, an unsteady gait, paralysis, and respiratory failure, which may lead to death.

The marine vertebrate that most commonly envenoms people is the stingray. Stingrays have one to four venomous spines on their tails, which they are able to flick like whips. Stingray envenomation causes severe pain; nausea, vomiting, rapid pulse, sweatiness, headache, fainting, seizures, paralysis, and death can also occur.

Utilizing a shuffling walk (dragging your feet) when walking in shallow water will prevent you from stepping on a stingray; you'll instead kick it from the side, which will irk it but not so much that it will sting you. It will most likely swim away without retaliation.

Diving Q&A

Q I kind of freak out sometimes. I'm concerned that if I went scuba diving I might panic and do something dangerous.

A If you are prone to panic attacks, or think you might flip out and do something truly irrational, then indeed you might want to limit your undersea exploration to snorkeling. As noted, you can kill yourself if you bolt to the surface while scuba diving.

Q I have a head cold. Can I dive?

A You shouldn't. Generally, when you have a head cold, your Eustachian tubes are clogged, such that you can't equalize the pressure in your middle ears. This will cause pain and possibly even rupture of the eardrums as you dive. If you can pop your ears—attempt to exhale through your nose while pinching it closed with your fingers and hearing a (nonpainful) pop in both ears—it's usually okay to dive.

Q I have bad allergies. Can I dive?

A Unless your allergies are well controlled, it's not a good idea. As with a head cold, allergies tend to clog your Eustachian tubes, causing pain on descent and ascent. For control of allergies, a long-acting medication, such as an intranasal steroid, is better than an oral one, the effectiveness of which may expire while you're diving, leading to pain on ascent.

Q I'm a woman in my childbearing years, and I'm sexually active and not using birth control. Should I dive?

A For obvious reasons, there will never be a controlled clinical trial on this issue, but both anecdotal reports and animal models suggest that fetal limb and cardiac defects are increased in those who scuba dive early in pregnancy; other problems have been linked to diving later in pregnancy. My advice is to either use reliable birth control or not scuba dive.

Q Is it true that menstruating women are at elevated risk of shark attack when they dive?

A No. Studies show no elevated risk.

Travel for Work

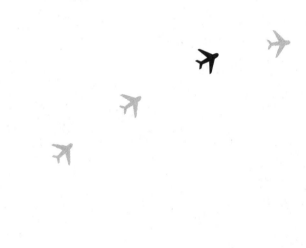

16

Corporate Travelers

The Bottom Line

As our economy becomes increasingly global, more corporations are sending employees abroad, often to low-income nations. Currently, about a quarter of international travel by US residents is work related. Although few of us can attain the proficiency at living within jets and hotels displayed by Ryan Bingham, the character played by George Clooney in the 2009 film *Up in the Air*, it is undeniable that certain practices will lead to a better quality of life while abroad.

The good news is that international travel for business is often profitable. Per the US Travel Association (www.ustravel.org), for every dollar spent on business travel, businesses saw an average of $9.50 in increased revenue and $2.90 in new profits. The bad news is that frequent international travel for work can take a toll on travelers.

A study of over 18,000 US business travelers published in 2017 found that those who were away from home more than six nights per month were more likely, relative to those who traveled less, to smoke, not exercise, have troubled sleep, and experience depression, anxiety, and alcohol dependence. Minor ailments are not rare among international business travelers. A study of 140 employees from western Canada's oil and gas industry who traveled internationally for work found that 74% had jet lag and 45% had travelers' diarrhea or other gastrointestinal complaints.

BEING A SHORT-TERM business traveler in no way exempts you from the usual pre-travel care, including immunizations, malaria prophylaxis, insect precautions, and caution regarding other threats, including motor vehicle accidents. Indeed, given that many business travelers are frequent visitors to low-income nations, these precautions are all the more important.

Business trips sometimes occur with very little advance notice. If you think future assignments might occur on short notice, rather than waiting until you have firm plans for a trip, it is reasonable to see a pre-travel provider in advance of a specific itinerary and state where you think it's likely you will go. Most pre-travel providers are fine working with a probable, as opposed to firm, itinerary. You can always consult via phone with your pre-travel provider if your actual trip varies from the trip you initially discussed, to determine whether or not you require additional pre-travel care.

Recall that influenza is more common in international travelers than in those who remain at home; also recall that near the equator it is a year-round illness. Immunization for influenza should be a high priority. Respiratory illness—influenza, upper respiratory illnesses, and so on—are the most common cause of loss of work by long-haul airline crews; diarrhea is the second most common cause.

Studies looking at the timing of travelers' diarrhea find that it's most common on the third day following arrival. Thus, even very short stay travelers are at risk.

Many cities have high levels of street crime. Travelers will want to discuss the risk of crime with hotel staff or coworkers familiar with the area.

It is prudent to read up on the customs and practices of those in the land you're visiting as these can affect protocol for meetings and social engagements with foreign colleagues. Some corporations develop guides for their employees who travel. Another reliable source for local customs is the Lonely Planet series of guidebooks.

Unlike vacationers, whose activities the first day or two at their destination may not be affected adversely by jet lag, people traveling for business can't afford to be groggy at high-stakes meetings. If possible, arrive early, giving yourself time to adjust.

Travelers should check with their employer regarding healthcare insurance while abroad, as well as emergency medical evacuation insurance. It seems reasonable, should the traveler not already have both, for the employer to pay for these.

Those who spend long durations—years—in TB-endemic nations should be screened for tuberculosis (TB) after their return. Screening for TB is also advised for those with exposure to work sites with elevated risk of TB: healthcare facilities, prisons, homeless shelters. Screening should occur eight weeks minimum after return.

As with nonbusiness travelers, sex with a new partner is not uncommon. As at home, if you have a new partner, safe sex is a must.

Corporate Travelers Q&A

Q I find travel stressful. Am I just a big wuss?

A Many people find travel stressful. A World Bank study that looked at post-travel insurance claims found that men who traveled overseas two or more times per year on business had a threefold elevated risk for submitting a claim for a psychiatric illness, such as depression or anxiety. Additionally, employees who remain abroad for a long duration may experience reverse culture shock as they reenter their own culture.

Q I have at least one chronic illness. I don't think I'm sufficiently fit to work in low-income nations. What should I do?

A On one hand, most travelers with most medical problems can visit most destinations. However, if you feel your medical condition precludes you from international travel, you should convey this to your pre-travel provider or regular physician. If that physician concurs, he or she can write a note to your employer, stating that you should not travel for medical reasons. Most employers will accept such a note and send someone else.

Legally, they have to: The Americans with Disabilities Act (ADA) offers protection to employees with chronic medical conditions. Employers may not require employees to engage in activities that present a significant threat to health.

Q I find that taking a malaria medication, such as doxycycline, for twenty-eight days after my trip to be a major pain.

A Use Malarone instead. You have to take it only for seven days after leaving the malaria-endemic area.

Q What if my host offers me something that I think could give me diarrhea? I don't want to be rude.

A It's a personal call, but my thought is that it would be unlikely that your host would give you something that was particularly high risk. Indeed, declining a particular meal could be seen as impolite. As I say, it's a personal call.

Q I've heard that my hosts in Country X drink like fish. The last person from my company to go there said he got completely sloshed with them at a business dinner.

A My thought is that it is indeed improvident to get bombed with your business associates. The phrase "It isn't good for me" suggests a medical condition that precludes you from joining them in their overindulgence. If it were me, I wouldn't feel too bad about saying, after two drinks (or none at all) that you've had enough. If only from a vantage point of business strategy, there may be benefits from remaining relatively sober as your new associates grow increasingly blotto.

Q I love my laptop and would not consider travel without it.

A Given that you and your laptop may go your separate ways during your trip, it is important that you not keep sensitive data (e.g., employee information with personal data) on it.

Also, you should not keep the sole copy of anything on your laptop. If a large project exists only on your laptop and it's stolen, you'll be blue. One safe location to keep documents is online (e.g., as an email attachment). Also, you can put sensitive information on a jump drive that you keep on your person in a secure location.

Q I spend a lot of time on jets. What can I do to minimize risks to health?
A See chapter 13.

Q I smoke. I can't smoke on jets. I might become really, really tense, or worse.
A Quit smoking. It's bad for you. In the meantime, consider use of the nicotine patch or nicotine gum, both of which, since 1996, are available in the US without a prescription.

Q Is food on jets safe?
A By and large, yes. This is fortunate. One hesitates to conjure a scenario in which every passenger on a jet has urgent diarrhea.

Q Clearly, if I'm having frequent diarrhea, I won't be effective at my work abroad. Is there anything I can do to absolutely minimize my risk of this?
A Yes. In addition to following safe food guidelines (see chapter 4), you can take rifaximin (Xifaxan) daily (available by prescription only). Rifaximin is a nonabsorbed antibiotic; the medication remains in your gut and reduces the risk of travelers' diarrhea. Being nonabsorbed, rifaximin has only very rare side effects. The dose for diarrhea prevention is one 200 mg tablet once or twice per day. (Unfortunately, currently in the US it's quite expensive.) Another option is taking Pepto-Bismol (see chapter 4).

Q   Is there anything else I can do to feel better when I'm
    jet-lagged?
A   Exercise is a beautiful thing. Many hotels have gyms; if they
    don't, walking is much better than nothing. Exercise causes
    your brain to release endorphins, which have favorable mood
    and energy effects. By and large, you'll feel better if you can
    get some exercise and worse if you only sit around all day.

Q   Hotel food is junky, and I gain weight when I travel.
A   Indeed, hotels seem to favor high-fat, high-sweet fare, and
    healthy eating can require deliberate planning. One lightweight
    option is prepackaged individual-serving oatmeal packets. Most
    hotel rooms have a coffeemaker; you can heat water in that and
    have a reasonably high fiber and safe breakfast or snack. (You
    can use tap water if it's heated to boiling.)

    A diet high in fruits and vegetables—ideal within high-
    income nations—is a tad problematic, as there is thought to
    be an elevated risk of travelers' diarrhea from consuming most
    produce. Short-term travelers particularly should avoid lettuce
    and other greens; long-term expats may want to consider a daily
    multivitamin.

Healthcare Workers

The Bottom Line

Increasingly, healthcare workers are volunteering to work in low-income nations. This mode of practice can, potentially, help people who would go without care but for volunteers, and it can be enormously satisfying to the healthcare worker. However, healthcare workers in low-resource settings are potentially exposed to a number of infectious diseases and other threats. Pre-travel planning and precautions while providing care can mitigate the risks.

Blood-borne Pathogens

In low-income nations the risk of occupational exposure to blood-borne pathogens is increased by the high prevalence of diseases spread by blood as well as the absence of the usual safety equipment and practices. Nonretracting fingerstick lancets and glass capillary tubes, both of which have transmitted HIV to medical workers, are commonly used to test for illnesses such as malaria. Routine protective gear, including gloves, gowns, masks, and goggles, are often not available.

Exacerbating this risk is the desire of some patients in low-income countries to receive at least one injection during a medical encounter. In Ghana, 80% to 90% of patients who visit medical clinics receive one or more injections per visit. Many patients may feel that if you haven't administered an injection, you haven't done anything. You may need to explain your rationale for not giving an injection to every patient; however, your explanation may be met with skepticism.

It is prudent to pack and transport personal protection gear—gloves, gowns, masks, and goggles—yourself. If a sharps container isn't available at your work site, create one using a soda can or plastic laundry detergent bottle. As at your usual work site, you should not recap needles.

If a needlestick injury occurs, note the source patient's region of origin, presenting complaints, and findings on physical exam. If possible, perform a rapid HIV test on the source patient; in lieu of that, obtain a blood sample for later testing. Wash the injury site thoroughly with warm water and soap. Avoid caustic antiseptics (e.g., bleach and povidone iodine), which can increase the risk of infection as a result of tissue injury and recruitment of inflammatory cells.

HEPATITIS B

The prevalence of chronic hepatitis B infection is high (greater than 8%) in China, Southeast Asia, the Pacific Basin (excluding Japan, Australia, and New Zealand), the Amazon Basin, sub-Saharan Africa, some regions in the Middle East, the central Asian Republics, and a few nations in Eastern Europe. Of the 350 million to 400 million people worldwide who are infected with hepatitis B, one-third live in China.

Regions with low endemicity (under 2%) include North America, western and northern Europe, Australia, and regions of South America. The rest of the world has intermediate levels (2%–8%) of chronic hepatitis B infection.

The risk of an unvaccinated person acquiring hepatitis B infection following a needlestick injury is 1% to 6% if the source is negative for hepatitis B e-antigen (HBeAg) and 22% to 30% if the source is positive for HBeAg.

Among individuals receiving the primary series of three doses of hepatitis B vaccine, 90% respond. Between 30% and 50% of those who don't respond to the primary series will respond to a repeat vaccination series. Before repeating the series, check antibody to hepatitis B core antigen and HBsAg to make sure you're not a chronic carrier. If you are large, a deep intramuscular injection with a longer needle may be required. If you are still seronegative (your antibody is below protective level) after two series of three doses of hepatitis B vaccine, there is no benefit to repeated doses of vaccine.

If you are a hepatitis B vaccine nonresponder and you sustain a needlestick injury, you should receive hepatitis B immunoglobulin both after the exposure and again at one month following the needlestick. The dose is 0.06 mg/kg IM. Hepatitis B immunoglobulin started within one week of exposure reduces risk of acquiring hepatitis B infection by about 75%.

HEPATITIS C

The prevalence of hepatitis C in the US is 0.8% to 1.2%. Worldwide it is 2% to 3%. The incidence is significantly higher in many countries in Africa and Asia. Egypt has the highest prevalence of hepatitis C, up to 20% in some regions. Egypt's high level of hepatitis C is thought to have been caused by the widespread practice of reusing needles during campaigns of parenteral treatment for schistosomiasis.

The risk of transmitting hepatitis C via needlestick injury is 1.8% per exposure, which is significantly lower than that for hepatitis B. Of those who do acquire infection, up to 20% resolve spontaneously. Following exposure, no prophylaxis is advised, but you should be monitored with HCV RNA testing for four to twelve weeks, which is the incubation period of hepatitis C, following the exposure.

Globally, about 37 million people are HIV-positive; only about 60% of these people are aware of their HIV status. Approximately 1.8 million infections occur per year. In many African nations the prevalence of HIV/AIDS is extremely high:

HIV Prevalence in Adults, Ages 15–49, 2016 (Estimate)

Swaziland	27%
Lesotho	25%
Botswana	22%
South Africa	19%
Namibia	14%
Mozambique	12%
Malawi	9%
Uganda	7%
Kenya	5%
Tanzania	5%

Source: World Factbook, US Central Intelligence Agency.

HIV can be transmitted by blood, semen, vaginal secretions, vomitus, breast milk, or pus from an HIV-positive person. Sweat, tears, saliva, and urine do not transmit HIV unless they are contaminated with blood. The risk of acquiring HIV infection following a needlestick injury from an HIV-positive source is lower than that for both hepatitis B and hepatitis C, 0.3%, or about 1 in 300. This risk can be markedly reduced by taking post-exposure prophylaxis (PEP). PEP is most effective if taken immediately following the exposure; in any event, it should be started within three days of exposure.

The HIV PEP regimen consists of emtricitabine/tenofovir (Truvada) and raltegravir (Isentress). The dose is 200 mg emtricitabine/ 300 mg tenofovir, one tablet per day, with raltegravir (Isentress) at a dose of 400 mg, one tablet twice per day, for twenty-eight days. The advised regimen is subject to change, so check the Centers for Disease Control (CDC) website (www.cdc.gov) for current recommendations. I often write a prescription for a few days of PEP regimen for healthcare workers who are planning to work abroad in areas with a high prevalence of HIV. I write for as little as two days of this for those who will work in large urban centers with rapid access to drugs and an airport, or for five days or more for those who will be more remote. The plan is for the healthcare worker to start the medications ASAP following exposure, then to obtain more medications with which to complete the twenty-eight-day series.

Inform your healthcare provider of the needlestick injury. Serologic testing for HIV, hepatitis B and C, and syphilis should be conducted immediately following the exposure, to establish a baseline, and again at three months following the exposure. HIV RNA should be checked if you develop a fever after exposure to an HIV-positive source. HIV RNA can be checked, if available, at two, six, twelve, and twenty-four weeks following a high-risk exposure.

VIRAL HEMORRHAGIC FEVER

Viral hemorrhagic fever (VHF), an acute febrile illness accompanied by a bleeding diathesis, is caused by four families of viruses: filoviruses (e.g., Ebola, Marburg), flaviviruses (e.g., yellow fever, dengue fever), arenaviruses (e.g., Lassa fever), and bunyaviruses (e.g., Crimean–Congo hemorrhagic fever, Rift Valley fever). Risk of exposure can be reduced by appropriate protective measures.

Although these illnesses are rare, with the exception of dengue fever, in those who visit endemic nations, they are frightening to the layperson and medical professional alike. (A friend told me, just prior to my first departure for East Africa, "Wouldn't go there myself. No sirree, there's something about *total liquefaction* of all your internal organs. . . .") Medical workers should know which viral hemorrhagic fevers are endemic to the area in which they will be working. Early diagnosis of this large group of illnesses can be difficult, as presentations vary widely. Hemorrhagic manifestations may include oozing at intravenous puncture sites, petechiae, purpura, large ecchymoses, or frank hemorrhage. Case fatality rates vary from under 1%, as with Rift Valley fever, to almost 90% with some outbreaks of Ebola. Specific diagnosis cannot be made clinically; diagnosis depends on detection of virus or virus antigens in serum, plasma, or whole blood.

In addition to spreading via exposure to blood, all viral hemorrhagic fevers, with the exception of dengue fever, can be spread by aerosols. Fortunately, person-to-person transmission of VHFs is rare. In the Zaire (now Democratic Republic of the Congo) 1995 Ebola epidemic, infections of healthcare workers occurred but lessened markedly after isolation precautions. The absence of personal protection equipment, along with the heat and humidity, can make adherence to isolation precautions a challenge.

Standard, contact, and droplet precautions should be utilized when dealing with patients with suspected VHF in both inpatient and outpatient settings. The World Health Organization (WHO) and CDC have developed pragmatic protocols of infection-control measures appropriate for low-resource settings, which they post on their respective websites (www.who.int, www.cdc.gov).

Following exposure, consultation with an infectious disease specialist for treatment or prophylaxis is prudent.

EBOLA OUTBREAK IN WEST AFRICA

Prior to the Ebola outbreak in West Africa in 2014 to 2016, outbreaks of Ebola were relatively small, the largest being the 2000 to 2001 outbreak in Uganda, in which 425 people were infected.

The Ebola outbreak of 2014 to 2016 was centered in Guinea, Sierra Leone, and Liberia and caused more than 11,000 deaths. The overall case-fatality rate was slightly above 70%; the case-fatality rate for those hospitalized with Ebola was some-where between 57% and 59%.

More than 500 healthcare workers in Guinea, Sierra Leone, and Liberia were killed by Ebola during this epidemic. Given the chronic shortage of healthcare professionals in these countries, the epidemic had a devastating effect on local healthcare systems.

Tuberculosis

Tuberculosis (TB) is common in low-income nations around the world. Although most TB remains sensitive to the usual anti-TB medications, both multidrug-resistant tuberculosis (MDR TB) and extensively drug-resistant tuberculosis (XDR TB) are on the rise. Half a million new cases of MDR TB were reported in 2015. About 9.5% of those infected with MDR TB have XDR TB. XDR TB has been reported in 117 countries.

Recognition of individuals with MDR and XDR TB is difficult in low-resource settings. Laboratory infrastructure, including the capacity to perform culture and sensitivity testing, may be limited or absent. Treatment for these infections is lengthy, with significant toxicity, and poor outcomes are common.

Nations of the former Soviet Union have the highest known prevalence of drug-resistant TB: 20% of all cases of TB in the former Soviet Union are MDR. China represents 25% of the global burden of drug-resistant TB; India accounts for more than 20%; many nations in Africa, Vietnam, Thailand, Korea, the Philippines, Peru, and Guatemala also have relatively high rates (more than 3%) of MDR.

In endemic areas, transmission of TB occurs not only in hospitals but also in other areas with relatively crowded conditions, including medical clinics, hospices, orphanages, and prisons. Although use of a fit-tested disposable filtering facepiece respirator is advised, few practitioners in low-resource settings utilize these. Thus, healthcare

DEFINITIONS: MDR TB AND XDR TB

Multidrug-resistant tuberculosis (MDR TB): tuberculosis resistant to both isoniazid (INH) and rifampin (RIF).

Extensively drug-resistant tuberculosis (XDR TB): MDR tuberculosis plus resistance to fluoroquinolones (a large group of broad-spectrum antibiotics) and a second-line injectable medication (kanamycin [Kantrex], amikacin [Amikin], or capreomycin [Capastat]).

workers should be screened regularly for TB, either via interferon gamma release assay (IGRA) or tuberculin skin testing (TST). IGRA is the more specific of the two types of screening. Screening with IGRA should be conducted at least two months after return. Screening with TST should be conducted no sooner than eight weeks after return.

Treatment of latent TB, which is by definition present when one has a positive IGRA or TST but no symptoms and a normal chest x-ray, is strongly recommended. Effective regimens include isoniazid (INH) daily for nine months, or rifampin (RIF) daily for four months. Treatment of latent tuberculosis after significant exposure to a region with a high prevalence of MDR or XDR tuberculosis is controversial. Some experts advise treatment with six to twelve months of either ethambutol (Myambutol) or pyrazinamide (Rifater) with either levofloxacin (Levaquin) or moxifloxacin (Avelox), after exposure to a region of high prevalence. Regular clinical and radiographic follow-up for twenty-four months is advised for those with likely MDR or XDR pathogens, whether or not treatment is initiated.

Should active tuberculosis develop, obtaining information regarding resistance should be obtained promptly. Determination of resistance, on a molecular level, can be performed at the CDC and some but not all US state health departments. Consultation with an expert is wise; specialists at the CDC's TB Centers of Excellence for Training, Education, and Medical Consultation are available for phone consults.

Healthcare personnel (and others with anticipated routine contact with at-risk sites, such as prisons or homeless shelters) should receive pre-travel screening for TB with either a two-step TST, in which those whose baseline TST is negative are retested one to three weeks after the first, or an IGRA. After travel, screening should be repeated. The TST should be performed eight to ten weeks after travel; the IGRA should be done at least eight weeks after travel.

Severe Respiratory Viral Infections

In the 2003 severe acute respiratory syndrome (SARS) pandemic, nosocomial transmission to healthcare workers was common. Avian influenza A (H5N1) is currently widespread in poultry and wild bird populations, causing infrequent human cases in Southeast Asia and the Middle East. The case-fatality rate is above 60%. Fortunately, human-to-human transmission is rare.

In 2009, a novel reassortment influenza virus subtype A (H1N1)—often referred to as swine flu—appeared in North America and spread worldwide. Known as pandemic flu (as opposed to the seasonal flu that occurs every year), it caused more than three hundred thousand confirmed cases and more than seventeen thousand deaths in more than two hundred countries. Relatively small outbreaks have occurred since then.

Transmission of SARS occurs predominantly via close interactions with infected people. During the pandemic, transmission to healthcare workers was more frequent in those performing certain procedures, including endotracheal intubation. Spread of infection to healthcare workers was markedly reduced following implementation of infection-control measures.

Influenza viruses are spread via large droplets, direct and indirect contact, and droplet nuclei. The degree to which transmission of influenza is airborne is controversial. In regions with high heat and humidity, direct contact may be a more important route of spread than inhalation.

Risk of transmission of many respiratory viruses, particularly influenza, is markedly reduced by washing your hands frequently with soap and water. In the absence of a source of clean water, alcohol-based hand sanitizer gels should be used. Protective clothing, including gloves, shoe covers, goggles, and face masks offer additional protection. The use of fitted high-efficiency particle-filtering N95 respirators is controversial. Use of surgical (nonfitted) masks may reduce risk of seasonal influenza. Most nosocomial respiratory infections are spread by droplets, thus standard precautions plus droplet precautions reduce risk.

In low-resource settings, precautions should focus on hand hygiene, contact precautions, respiratory protection when indicated, and use of personal protection equipment (PPE) that offers protection against pathogens spread via respiratory aerosols, particularly during procedures at risk of generating aerosols, including intubation.

Following large-scale disasters, the CDC often posts announcements and advisories regarding widespread respiratory infections on its web page with specific advice for healthcare workers, as with its "Announcement: Guidance for Relief Workers and Others Traveling to Haiti for Earthquake Response," which was posted following the 2010 earthquake in Port-au-Prince, Haiti.

It is a proven medical fact that the IQ of medical providers plummets when they attempt to care for themselves. If you sustain an exposure or become ill, consult with another healthcare professional.

Road Traffic Accidents

As with tourists and business travelers, the greatest threat to healthcare workers is not infectious diseases but road traffic accidents. A 1985 study that looked at the deaths of Peace Corps Volunteers over a twenty-one-year period found that 70% of the 185 deaths of volunteers were caused by unintentional injury, almost half of which were due to motor vehicle accidents. Motorcycles caused 12% of all deaths and 33% of all motor vehicle fatalities. The Peace Corps saw a marked reduction in the deaths of its personnel when a policy that forbade travel by motorcycle for the great majority of their volunteers was instituted. (Drowning accounted for 18% of the unintentional injury deaths.) A follow-up study that looked at the deaths of Peace Corps Workers between 1984 and 2003 found a lower overall rate of death, with motor vehicle accidents remaining the most common cause of death.

Disaster Response: Lessons Learned

For a thirteen-year period (2004 to 2017), I served as a medical officer on the International Medical-Surgical Response Team-West (IMSuRT-West; now named the Trauma and Critical Care Team [TCCT]), a US federal disaster response team based in Seattle. My deployments on this team included New Orleans following Hurricane Katrina, the 2007 wildfires in San Diego, and Port-au-Prince, Haiti, following the 2010 earthquake.

LESSONS THAT I'VE LEARNED

1. An effective command system is paramount. Incident Command System (ICS) should be utilized. Developed by California firefighters in the 1970s, ICS mandates a number of practices, including that the overall Incident Commander is on site, not situated in a distant office; that different players (e.g., military, police, health responders) use a common terminology; and that a limited number of personnel report to any one supervisor. The more I responded to disasters, the more I admired ICS's many virtues.

2. Generally speaking, you can accomplish much more as a member of a team than you can as a solo operator. During my team's deployments, we were effective only because we deployed with a variety of nonmedical staff, including logistics, communications, and security personnel. Indeed, as a lone practitioner in a

disaster setting, you may yourself end up needing care and become a net liability.

3. The time to become involved in disaster relief is not immediately following a disaster but during a relative lull. Credentialing of medical personnel is not a rapid process, and it is difficult to impossible immediately following a disaster. A panoply of organizations provide care following disasters; one is the International Federation of Red Cross and Red Crescent Societies (www.ifrc.org).

4. What you have is what you have. You can't assume that anything will be available at the site of a disaster. Food, water, medical supplies, other—all should be transported with you.

5. Communications should be redundant. In disasters, both landlines and cell phones tend to fail. Use of ham radio or walkie-talkies may make communication possible.

6. Transport of the injured by ground following a disaster may not be possible. Transport by air (e.g., helicopters) may be the only method of transporting the ill and injured. Designating an area to serve as a helicopter landing zone, and having an intact form of communications (see truism 5) are essential to coordinate transport by air.

7. Most of the ill may be ill not as a direct effect of the disaster but from the abrupt withdrawal of usual medical care. Plans to care for the chronically ill should be made.

8. The rules change; flexibility is essential. Documentation is markedly reduced. You may need to establish a hospice for those who will fare poorly regardless of medical care so that you can focus your efforts on those with a more favorable prognosis. You may need to transport grossly unstable patients via ambulance or helicopter. It is the opposite of business as usual; you will have to change your practices on a regular basis as resources and needs ebb and flow.

9. The US military has helicopters, drugs and other medical supplies, communications equipment and procedures, and capable

personnel. I have been struck by the professionalism of the military personnel with whom I've worked following disasters. If it's an option, networking with the US military is often helpful.

10. A final observation: Most people rise to the situation. As a rule, the victims of disasters wait in line and say thank you; medical providers work extremely long hours, under arduous conditions, without complaint. I have witnessed much more benevolent and noble behavior, among those affected by disasters and medical providers alike, than people acting poorly. Indeed, my work with communities affected by disasters has made me rather optimistic about human nature.

TRAUMA AND CRITICAL CARE TEAM

There are three Trauma and Critical Care Teams (TCCTs) in the US: TCCT-West, based at Harborview Medical Center in Seattle; TCCT-East, based at Massachusetts General Hospital in Boston; and TCCT-South, based at Jackson Memorial Hospital in Miami. There are 55 DMATs (Disaster Medical Assistance Teams) in the US. Many states have one; larger states, such as California, have several. Both TCCTs and DMATs are under the National Disaster Medical System (NDMS), which is under the Department of Health and Human Services. TCCTs are configured as full surgical field hospitals; DMATs serve more as outpatient clinics. In addition to medical staff, each team has a number of logistics, communications, safety, and security personnel. Both TCCTs and DMATs respond to both domestic and foreign disasters.

Healthcare Worker Q&A

Q I have expired medications. Should I take those to distribute to my patients?

A My advice is that you hold off on taking expired medications abroad. For openers, even in low-income countries, many people can read, and your patients may very well read the bottle or blister pack and ask why you're dispensing an expired medication. You wouldn't give an expired medication to your patient in an affluent nation; I think it's hard to defend doing so in a low-resource setting.

Q **I only have a few days off here and there. Can I be an effective medical provider if I only work abroad for a brief while?**

A For a few specific conditions, such as cleft palate and cataracts, short-term intervention—that is, surgery—is indisputably of benefit. However, the great majority of medical problems, in low-income nations as in the affluent world, are of a chronic nature. It is difficult or impossible to offer benefit for chronic problems with care offered over a brief duration only. It takes time to learn the lay of the land; it takes time to learn what works and what doesn't in a given setting. As a general rule, the more you work in a single locale, the more effective you'll be. If you work abroad on a regular basis, I advise you to return to the same area.

Q **Can I assume that generally agreed-upon ethics in my land of origin are identical worldwide?**

A No. Ethical norms vary widely worldwide. In Ethiopia, for example, an unfavorable prognosis is told not to a patient but to a family member or close friend who will inform the patient at a setting deemed appropriate. It's a good idea to study the ethical norms of the region in which you'll be working.

Other Considerations

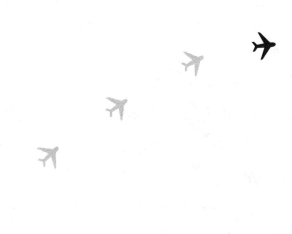

The Medical Kit

The Bottom Line

You can't pack everything you might possibly need, but carrying a few key medical supplies is prudent. International travelers must always be conscious of the weight of their luggage—less is better—but a small medical kit can come in handy.

A MEDICAL KIT typically contains over-the-counter and prescription medications and supplies and equipment such as bandages, a thermometer, and tweezers, but don't forget to bring sunblock and vision care supplies as well.

Medications

Keep all medications, both prescription and over-the-counter, in their original containers. Unlabeled pills in an envelope or plastic bag can draw scrutiny at Customs. Carry all medications in your carry-on luggage, not in checked luggage, in case you and your checked luggage go to separate continents. Check out the Transportation Security Administration (TSA) website (www.tsa.gov) for rules and travel tips. As of this writing, the TSA limit on liquids, gels, and pastes at screening is no more than 3.4 ounces (100 milliliters) in one bag that's no bigger than one quart (which is bigger than a sandwich bag but smaller than a big freezer bag).

Acetaminophen (Tylenol) and/or aspirin and/or ibuprofen (Advil, Motrin)
Diphenhydramine (Benadryl)
Loperamide (Imodium)

Antibiotic cream (e.g., Polysporin)
Antifungal cream (e.g., Lamisil)
Steroid cream (e.g., hydrocortisone 1%)

These depend on your destination and itinerary. For short-term travelers to popular resorts, the only prescription medication I'd recommend that you carry is an antibiotic for travelers' diarrhea. If you will be in a malaria area, carry an antimalarial (see chapter 3).

If you need medications intermittently (e.g., for migraine headaches, asthma, or bladder infections), you should assume that whatever condition you have will flare while you're abroad, and pack appropriate medications.

Upper respiratory infections are common in international travelers. Consider packing whichever over-the-counter medications (e.g., decongestant, throat lozenges, cough syrup) you find of benefit.

Constipation—possibly brought on by prolonged sitting during jet travel and reduced fluid intake—is common in travelers. You may want to pack and take a fiber product such as psyllium (e.g., Metamucil) during travel.

Medical Stuff

Thermometer

Pair of fine-point tweezers (for splinter removal)

Adhesive strip bandages

Padded adhesive for feet for blister prevention or treatment (e.g., Moleskin or Molefoam)

Iodine tablets for water purification

Oral rehydration solution powder for infants or elderly travelers

Sunblock (see below)

Bag Balm (I don't travel with this myself, but I've heard and read that Bag Balm, developed for cow's udders, is an excellent, inexpensive topical antibiotic.)

DEET-based insect repellent or picaridin 20% for skin, and permethrin for clothing (see chapter 3). For trips under six weeks, apply permethrin prior to travel and leave it at home.

SUNBLOCK

Sunblock is important. Direct sunlight at the equator is roughly equivalent to a tanning bed: If you're fair, twenty minutes will give you a rosy glow, one hour can cause blisters, six hours can land you in the hospital with second-degree burns. The SPF (sun protection factor) should be at least 30.

Sunblock should be applied at least half an hour prior to exposure to the sun so that it can be absorbed by your skin. It's fine to apply sunblock and insect repellent together. When applying both, apply the sunblock first, give it fifteen minutes or so for your skin to absorb it, then apply the repellent. If you're swimming, a waterproof brand of sunblock is best.

Avoid the combination bug repellent and sunscreen preparations; they tend to contain too much of one and too little of the other.

VISION CARE

Something that is virtually weight free is a copy of your prescription for eyeglasses or contacts. You can get this from your optician, optometrist, or ophthalmologist. Glasses seem to have a propensity for being sat on, stepped on, or otherwise destroyed during international travel. Most large cites will have an optician who can re-create your eyeglasses for minimal cost. Consider taking an old pair of glasses as a backup.

Note: Contact lens wearers should use clean water (e.g., bottled or boiled, then cooled) for handwashing before handling lenses and for rinsing hard (gas permeable) lenses.

NEEDLES

If you require injections or infusions of medications on a regular basis, pack an adequate number of sterile needles and syringes for your trip. Travelers should carry a letter from the prescribing clinician, on letterhead stationary, stating the purpose of needles and syringes. In the US, Transportation Security Administration (TSA) allows unused syringes when accompanied by injectable medication. Travelers must declare these items to security officers at security checkpoints for inspection. TSA allows used syringes when carried in a hard-surface container.

MEDICAL DOCUMENTATION

Phone numbers and e-mail addresses of your doctors and health insurance contacts back home

List of medications with doses

List of allergies

Wallet card that your emergency air evacuation company gives you when you sign up, with its contact information

Consider e-mailing this information to yourself, so that you can access it should you lose all your belongings.

FOR WOMEN TRAVELERS

Women may want to pack supplies for menstruation, medications to treat bladder and vaginal infections, and emergency contraception. (See chapter 7.)

Medical Kit Q&A

Q **What about a snakebite kit?**

A If you are bitten by a snake, seek medical care immediately. The old cowboy strategy of making a cut with a knife at the site of the snakebite, then attempting to suck out the poison is not recommended. Dr. David Warrell, emeritus professor of tropical medicine at the University of Oxford, an authority on treatment of bites of venomous snakes, states that the less you do at the bite site (other than to wash it with soap and water), the better.

Those at highest risk of venomous snakebite in the tropics are those with occupational exposure (e.g., farmers). Risk is low in tourists.

Q **Should I take extra medicines so that I can share them with people I meet?**

A No. Your heart may be in the right place, but unless you are a physician and plan on taking detailed histories and performing physical exams and appropriate laboratory testing, you can easily do more harm than good. A few brief examples: You think a man has a head cold, and you share your penicillin. He's allergic to penicillin. He dies. You share an anti-malarial, primaquine, with a woman whom you think has malaria. You neglect to first check to see if she is G6PD-deficient, which she is. The primaquine kills her. You think a boy has travelers' diarrhea, and you share your antibiotic. He has appendicitis, and he dies. You get the idea. Even nonprescription medications have the potential for significant harm if misused. There is a reason that medical school and residency require, at a minimum, seven years.

Q I'm working abroad for years. Can I have relatives or friends mail me my personal medications from the US?

A Medications mailed between nations are often delayed at Customs for a very long time or are refused entry. The most reliable method of transporting prescription medications between countries is with a person, ideally the person for whom they are prescribed. Each should be transported in the original container in which it was dispensed from the pharmacy, and each should be labeled with the patient's name, prescribing physician, and pharmacy. For large amounts of medications (e.g., one year's worth or more) consider obtaining a letter from the prescribing physician detailing the medical conditions for which the medication(s) have been prescribed.

19

After Your Trip

The Bottom Line

Depending on where you've traveled, how long you've been gone, and what you've done, you may want to undergo a few screening tests after your return.

Post-Trip Q&A

Q I just returned from a trip to low- and/or middle-income nations, and I feel fine. Do I need any testing?
A It depends.

Q It depends on what?
A Primarily on the duration of your travels.

Q I was in Acapulco for a week. Do I need any screening?
A No.

Q Say I was there for years.
A Then you might consider a couple of tests. For anyone who spends years in a TB-endemic country, a test for latent tuberculosis is advised. Two tests are available: (1) the purified protein

derivative (PPD; skin test, also called tuberculin skin test [TST]) and (2) the interferon gamma release assay (IGRA, e.g., QuantiFERON-TB Gold, or T-Spot.*TB*), which involves a blood draw. The PPD is performed at least eight weeks after exiting the at-risk location. A medical provider places a bit of fluid under the skin of your forearm, then you return to that clinic forty-eight to seventy-two hours later to have the test read. If after the PPD is placed a bump of sufficient size appears, your test will be read as positive and a few months of an anti-TB medicine (e.g., isoniazid) will be recommended. Similarly, for those testing positive with an IGRA, isoniazid or another medication for TB for several months is advised.

The PPD is preferred for children under age 5. The IGRA is the preferred test for those who have received bacille Calmette-Guerin (BCG), a vaccine for TB.

Screening for latent TB is also advised for those who have traveled for shorter durations but have had exposure to at-risk populations, such as healthcare facilities, refugee camps, or prisons.

TUBERCULOSIS: LATENT VS. ACTIVE

Tuberculosis (TB) is a bacterial illness that is common in low-income nations around the world. Spread by coughing or speaking, TB can infect any organ in the body, but 90% of infections are pulmonary.

Clinicians differentiate between active and latent TB:

Latent TB: Live TB bacteria in the body, but no illness, no symptoms. People with latent TB are not contagious.

Active TB: Active infection, with symptoms. For example, the symptoms of pulmonary TB are cough for longer than three weeks, fever, and weight loss. People with active TB are contagious.

Screening for latent TB is advised for at-risk persons because about 10% of people with latent TB, over the course of their lives, will progress to active TB, which is life threatening. Taking a course of an anti-TB medication will markedly reduce the risk of progression from latent to active TB.

The PPD generally becomes positive four to ten weeks after an exposure; the IGRA usually becomes positive four to seven weeks after an exposure but can take longer.

Q What else?

A Long-duration (over one year) travelers to low- or middle-income countries can consider getting a stool test. Basically, you give a lab some of your stool, which is then examined under the microscope for worm eggs and other things that ought not be there. Anything they can find can be eliminated with the right drug. In addition, your stool may be tested with a polymerase chain reaction (PCR) test such as BioFire Film Array Gastrointestinal Panel, which tests for twenty-two bacteria, protozoa, and viruses. Research on the benefits of testing stool in those without symptoms after travel is sparse.

Q Worms! Give the lab some of my poop? Gross!

A Well, yes.

Q I hope you're finished.

A There is another test or two to consider, such as the test for the disease called schistosomiasis (also called bilharzia). It is transmitted in contaminated bodies of fresh water throughout the continent of Africa and a few other places.

Q I was only in Mexico.

A It's not in Mexico. For those who have been in any body of fresh water in Africa or other region endemic for schistosomiasis, a blood test is advised, at least six to eight weeks after potential exposure. Anyone who tests positive receives a single dose of a drug called praziquantel.

Q I swam in fresh water. I feel fine. Should I be tested for leptospirosis?

A Screening of returned travelers without symptoms for leptospirosis is not advised. Usual symptoms of leptospirosis are fever, headache, chills, muscle aches, vomiting, and jaundice.

Q Are you finished?

A Almost. Those who have had exposure to soil that may have been contaminated with human feces—as from frequently walking barefoot outdoors—should consider a blood test for *Strongyloides*, a parasitic infection

Q I had sex with a new partner while abroad. Should I be tested for anything?

A Yes, you should be screened for a number of sexually transmitted infections (STIs) and blood-borne infections: chlamydia and gonorrhea, HIV, syphilis, and hepatitis B and C. This is all the more important if you had sex without a condom.

Q What if I'm sick when I return home?

A If you feel unwell after your trip, you want to see a physician who sees returned ill travelers regularly. There is no board certification for travel or tropical medicine, but one marker of travel-health savvy is a Certificate of Knowledge in Clinical Tropical Medicine & Travelers' Health from the American Society of Tropical Medicine and Hygiene (ASTMH). The ASTMH gives a rigorous exam every two years on both pre-travel and post-travel medicine; those who pass are awarded this certificate. The International Society of Travel Medicine (ISTM) regularly conducts exams and issues Certificates of Travel Health; this exam covers pre-travel care only.

While traveling in low- and middle-income nations, travelers should keep in mind that diagnostic tests may not be performed with the accuracy we are accustomed to in the US and other high-income nations. I see many travelers who have received a diagnosis of malaria while traveling in Africa and elsewhere. Well over half, when I test them, do not have and have not recently had malaria. Often these travelers took their preventative medicines for malaria as they were advised to do. In these people, malaria is very rare. If you are taking an appropriate medication to prevent malaria and you develop fever, other causes, including dengue fever and influenza, are more likely. Often travelers are told that the local malaria is resistant to doxycycline or whichever medication the traveler is on. Unfortunately, this has prompted some travelers to stop their preventative medication, at which point they may develop malaria on top of whatever illness first prompted them to seek medical care.

Additional Tips

The Bottom Line

- Quite often, spending less money, not more, will increase your enjoyment while abroad.
- Travel with a guidebook.
- Hire guides.
- Avoid chain restaurants and chain hotels.
- Don't complain.
- Be a responsible traveler.

MANY PEOPLE TRAVEL to enter into a state that could be called the travel epiphany, or what Spalding Gray, in his monologue *Swimming to Cambodia*, called the "perfect moment." The perfect moment is that instant during which your soul says "Ahhh!" as though it had an itchy back and someone were scratching it. Something previously jumbled aligns, and you are content in a way that is difficult to articulate.

Do not wait until you are at the mountaintop, or the temple, or the waterfall, before you are open to having your touristic epiphany. Tourism is not geographically determined; it is determined by your attitude. You can see amazing things at a bus station or in someone's backyard. You will have travel epiphanies not in proportion to your environs but to the extent that you are open to them. (For those with an interest in the sociology of tourism, *The Tourist: A New Theory of the Leisure Class* by Dean MacCannell, a sociologist at the University of California, Davis, is a fascinating and insightful book.)

I do not know why Herman Melville, in *Moby-Dick*, wrote, "Lima, the strangest, saddest city thou can'st see." I attended a nine-week tropical medicine course in Lima and found it charming and commodious. But nonetheless big cities are not known for their propensity for extending a welcoming hand to newcomers.

The link between travel and mood has been recognized for some time. Strabo (63 BC–24 AD), in his *Geography*, wrote, "The country [Albania] produces some venomous reptiles, as scorpions and tarantulas. These tarantulas cause death in some instances by laughter, in others by grief and a longing to return home." Just as parents should pack teddy bears and blankies for their children, so should adults carry some small object able to transport them to their happy and calm places. A journal, novel, or a music player can soothe a frayed psyche.

Realize that when something unexpected occurs, it may turn out to be the best part of your trip. There is an interval of time—call it the event-to-anecdote interval—between the occurrence of whatever odd surprise happens to you and your realization that this turn of events, although it may delay or change your plans, is in fact a travel anecdote that you can share upon your return. Suppose your bus breaks down in the middle of nowhere, and you have to ask a farmer if you can sleep on his floor, and of course he says yes, and when you wake up there are kittens between your legs and four children are watching you like you're a TV program. Now, this may not be how you would choose to greet the day, but when you get home and relate this tale you will be the envy of your social set. You risked serendipity and were rewarded.

Here are a few general rules to recall while under duress:

- Most people are nice.
- Most people are sane.
- Most people are honest.

Mental Health Q&A

Q **I'm just divorced/fired/otherwise and in crisis. I want to get away from it all. Is going to a low-income nation a good call?**

A Probably not. I'm a big proponent of visiting the less wealthy nations, but I would not say that travel therein is low stress; on the contrary, travel in a crowded, noisy, unfamiliar country at times can cause quite high stress. This is fine if you're starting off in a relatively placid state of mind, but if you're already in turmoil before you leave, I doubt that you'll find the peace of mind you're looking for. My advice: Stay home or travel to some orderly land, such as any nation in Western Europe.

Other Tips

Generally speaking, your experiences will be interesting in inverse proportion to the amount of money you spend. If you stay in a ritzy hotel in a big city, you will be very comfortable and will have absolutely nothing interesting to relate when you return. (You think people back home want to hear about how upset you got that morning when room service was so slow? Or the fuzziness of those slippers?) But if you take a bus trip—particularly if your bus breaks down—why, folks will be on the edge of their seats. You can stay at a swank place and have breakfast by yourself at a linen-covered table, or, for a twentieth of the price, you can stay at a hostel where you'll be thrown together, in courtyards and at mealtimes, with other guests. This is good if they are interesting and bad if they are not, but either way there is more likelihood of wonderfulness occurring at the hostel.

- *Buy a guidebook* prior to your trip and read it.
- *Learn a few words of the language of the countries you visit.* Becoming fluent is probably not realistic for most of us, but locals will appreciate even inept efforts to speak their language. Before I traveled to East Africa, I memorized perhaps a hundred words of Swahili and learned that the word for newspaper is *gazeti*; I realized that this told me not only what language that word is borrowed from but the approximate time (Victorian era) of the borrowing.
- *Hire guides.* I've never regretted hiring a guide. However, lest you think that all guides are perfect, allow me to share an anecdote told to me by Dr. C., one of my colleagues. He and his wife flew into the Mexico City airport with the intent of climbing Popocatepetl, a nearby volcano (17,800 feet [5,425 meters]). They were approached by a guide at the airport. Popocatepetl? No problem— the guide was intimate with its every route. However, a couple of days later, they were not far from the Tlamacas Lodge at 12,950 feet (3,950 meters) when their guide (who in retrospect did seem a little portly for a mountain guide) got lost *and* had an asthma attack. Being a family practice doctor, Dr. C. abandoned his climb, took care of his guide, and descended with him. I do not believe that Dr. C. and his wife ever did manage to climb Popo.

But this is the only story like this that I've heard—the vast majority of guides will enhance your travels. Exhibit A: Mark Twain. In *Innocents Abroad* and his writings on Hawaii, we read that the first thing he did in a new town was to hire a guide. If you hire guides, you are following in a long and honorable practice. Also by hiring a guide, there is a fair chance that your tourist dollar is going to the local economy.

If I think about the ten most recent guides I've hired, all ten have been wonderful. I saw places I wouldn't have seen without them. Mr. Liu, an elderly man who approached me on the Bund in Shanghai, took me into banks with vast marble columns and told me in some detail why these columns were magnificent. After twenty minutes he asked, "Would you like a rest?" and I replied, "What do you think?" "Good idea!" he said, and we sat on a park bench and had a most amiable chat.

- *Get off the bus/train/jet/boat.* Although views are wonderful and it's fun to watch the scenery go by, you will invariably get a better feel for any land outside of your transport vehicle. The most memorable aspects of my trip to the Copper Canyon of Mexico were the day hikes I took from Batopilas, a small village at the bottom of one of the canyons.

- *Do not complain.* Try this: Make a vow to yourself that not once while abroad are you going to complain. Complain internally—but try to keep your lip zipped if you're only going to bellyache about how miserable you are. Try to impress your traveling companions with your stoicism. Anyone can complain, but to keep your attitude sunny when the jet is cancelled, the taxi driver gets lost, the waiter brings something totally unrelated to what you think you ordered, and it's preternaturally hot and you're sleepy—that's behavior that will boost your status with traveling companions. If it's hot, if the bus isn't going anywhere, if the restaurant service is slow—keep mum. That's the way it is. You want snappy service? Go to a McDonald's in your home town.

- *Avoid the chains.* I admit that, buffeted by diffident or calamitous foreign land, familiar chains—McDonald's, Starbucks, and so on—can call out to you like the Sirens. Furthermore, I will not claim that I've never succumbed to their appeal. My wife and I, on our honeymoon, once ducked into a Kentucky Fried Chicken restaurant in Bangkok just to sit in its air conditioning for a while. But more of your tourist dollar will go to the local economy if you patronize businesses owned and run by locals.

- *Keep a journal.* You might think you will never forget that on Tuesday you visited Chichicastenango, then on Thursday you took a bus to Huehuetenango. But shortly after your trip, if you are like most of us, the names will blur and fade from your memory. Plus when you write to that tall Dane who studies Joyce whom you sat next to on the bus, you can mention in your letter (feigning an excellent memory) that you recall his love of stinky cheeses.

- *Hide your wristwatch in your carry-on* on your flight out. It can be surprisingly difficult, at first, to live without your wristwatch, but after a few days most people enjoy a state of lessened time awareness. And—for the truly bold—consider switching off your smartphone.

The Responsible Traveler

Travelers need to remain cognizant of the fact that they exert a huge impact on the peoples and lands that they visit. Dr. Irmgard Bauer, a researcher at James Cook University in Australia who studies the impact of tourists on the regions they visit, states that she can think of more negative than positive examples. An influx of tourists' cash often causes inflation, which decreases locals' buying power. Most of the money that tourists spend in rural areas does not stay in those regions but is funneled toward large, urban-based corporations.

Nonetheless, she has several suggestions for travelers to destinations outside high-income nations:

- Use local businesses rather than multinational corporations.
- Respect local customs. For example, if women are thought improper if they show their legs, don't wear shorts or a short skirt. It isn't your role to enlighten the world, at least not by what you wear. The Lonely Planet guidebooks usually carry well-informed sections detailing what is appropriate and what is not in terms of clothes, tipping, and so on.
- Don't give money to strangers. Michael McColl, director of communications for The Ethical Traveler, a San Francisco-based nonprofit, states, "Begging is not natural behavior for most cultures. . . . They probably learned it from other travelers before you—travelers who were not thinking through and taking responsibility for their actions." Rather than randomly giving money to strangers, better

to donate to a community organization—a nonprofit, a church, or a school. Or, after your return, find and support an organization that serves the community you visited.

- Don't give handouts to children. It's tempting, but as McColl explained, "It could condition them to do it again, perhaps becoming more aggressive in doing so in the future." Instead, consider giving items to parents, or teachers, or community leaders. Prior to your trip you can research the needs of a community.

And here are a few thoughts on ethics and courtesy:
- Leave a bit of money for the person who cleans your hotel room.
- Don't litter even if everyone else does.
- Do not tell people you're going to mail them copies of photos unless you will.
- If you are a student or researcher, share the results of your study with the people you are studying.

Is Everything Getting Worse?

Some say that foreign aid and medical interventions in low-income nations are pointless, that everything is getting worse, that the poor will always be poor, so why bother? But virtually every metric on global health says the opposite. Global childhood mortality has been reduced by 50% over the past twenty-five years. During the first half of the twentieth century, there were about two million deaths per year from malaria; due to control efforts, this was reduced to 429,000 deaths in 2015. In 1980 measles killed 2.6 million people; in 2015 this was reduced to 134,000—a 95% reduction. The number of people living in extreme poverty—earning less than $1.25 per day at 2005 prices—declined from 1.9 billion in 1990 to 1.2 billion in 2010. As recently as 1967, two million people were killed by smallpox; since then it has been eradicated from the planet.

As Stephen Pinker discusses in his 2012 book *The Better Angels of Our Nature: Why Violence Has Declined*, violence continues to decline worldwide. Consider the "stable" Roman Empire. Thirty-four out of forty-nine Roman emperors were killed by guards, high officials, or members of their family.

I'm not saying everything is rosy. Global climate change is an ongoing reality. There remain extreme disparities between people with money and those without. But most big trends are favorable. Global health efforts—by the World Health Organization (WHO), governmental foreign aid, and organizations including the Bill and Melinda Gates Foundation—have markedly improved global health in recent years. It may satisfy an apocalyptic narrative—or someone's political agenda—to state that everything is getting worse (and that foreign aid doesn't work), but it's just not so.

RESOURCES FOR GLOBAL TRAVELERS

For those desirous of more in-depth information on travel health, the CDC *Yellow Book: Health Information for International Travel* is an excellent resource, and as with every other topic known to humankind, there is a vast array of info regarding travel health on the internet. I've listed some high-yield sites here.

Print Resources

MEDICAL PUBLICATIONS

An extremely useful book for travelers and medical providers alike is the CDC's *Yellow Book: Health Information for International Travel* (commonly known as the Yellow Book), which is published every two years. It's available free online (www.cdc.gov; click on "Travelers' Health"), or you can order the print edition online or from your local bookseller.

A manual for those who want a more detailed description of tropical illnesses is *The Travel and Tropical Medicine Manual,* 5th edition (Elsevier, 2016), edited by myself and Drs. Elaine C. Jong and Paul S. Pottinger. Although primarily aimed at medical personnel, much of this will be comprehensible to the interested layperson.

An excellent text for medical personnel is *Travel Medicine,* 3rd edition, edited by Drs. Jay S. Keystone, David O. Freedman, Phyllis E. Kozarsky, Bradley A. Connor, and Hans D. Nothdurft (Mosby, 2013). For those venturing to high altitudes, Dr. Stephen Bezruchka's *Altitude Illness: Prevention and Treatment,* 2nd edition (Mountaineers Books, 2005), is readable, pragmatic, short, and inexpensive. Prevention and treatment of altitude illness are discussed in some detail in an article by A. M. Luks, S. E. McIntosh, C. K. Grissom, P. S. Auerbach, G. W. Rodway, R. B. Schoene, K. Zafren, and P. H. Hackett: "Wilderness Medical Society Practice Guidelines for the Prevention and Treatment of Acute Altitude Illness: 2014 Update," *Wilderness and Environmental Medicine*, vol. 25, number 4, suppl., pp. S4–S14 (2014, December).

NONMEDICAL PUBLICATIONS

The People's Guide to Mexico, 4th edition, by Carl Franz and Lorena Havens, edited by Steve Rogers and Felisa Churpa Rosa Rogers (Rick Steves, 2012), is so good that you should consider reading it even if you're not going to Mexico. Amazingly, this travel book mentions very few specific locations. It is about Mexico as a whole, and it is much more informative than the usual guidebooks as a result. Also, the authors' steadfast refusal to mention specific towns conveys the message that every place in Mexico, with the right attitude, is worthy of a visit. The museums and ruins aren't truer or realer—they're just more popular.

Online Resources

The Centers for Disease Control and Prevention (CDC), based in Atlanta, Georgia, is the US government's primary agency that advises US citizens regarding medical preparations for international travel. The agency's website (www.cdc.gov; click on button "Travelers' Health") provides detailed descriptions of all pertinent infectious diseases, with suggested preventative measures. Data are searchable by geographic region or specific disease. The information is top-notch and updated frequently. This is an excellent place to begin your pre-travel health preparations.

Similarly, the World Health Organization (WHO) maintains an excellent website (www.who.org) with up-to-date health information for international travelers.

The US State Department maintains a list of countries that Americans are advised to avoid (www.state.gov). Click the "Travel & Business" tab, then "Travel Warnings." Additionally, the State Department's "Background Notes" provide overviews of countries' land, people, history, government, political conditions, economy, and foreign relations.

Associations

Founded in 1960, the International Association for Medical Assistance to Travelers (IAMAT) is a Canada-based nonprofit organization that advises travelers about health risks and appropriate pre-travel measures. IAMAT also maintains a list of English-speaking physicians around the world who have trained in North America or Europe and who have agreed to treat IAMAT members. IAMAT personnel regularly inspect clinics to make sure they maintain high standards. (I accompanied Ms. Assunta Uffer-Marcolongo, president of IAMAT, on one of her inspection trips to China, and I can attest that she is thorough!) Website: www.iamat.org; tel. 716-754-4883.

If you are in a medically related field, two key organizations are the International Society of Travel Medicine (ISTM; www.istm.org) and the American Society of Tropical Medicine and Hygiene (ASTMH; www.astmh.org). ISTM, which was founded in 1978 and has more than thirty-five hundred members in more than a hundred countries, is more clinically based; ASTMH is more research oriented.

The Association for Safe International Road Travel (ASIRT) promotes global road safety through education and advocacy. The organization's website (www.asirt.org) lists a wide array of information and strategies to reduce risk.

Other organizations include the Wilderness Medical Society (WMS; http://wms.org), which has greater emphasis on outdoor sports, including backpacking and mountain climbing, and the UK-based Royal Society of Tropical Medicine and Hygiene (RSTMH; http://rstmh.org).

Two helpful sites regarding traveling with medications are the US Department of State Overseas Security Advisory Counsel (OSAC) website at https://www.osac.gov/pages/contentreportdetails.aspx ?cid=17386 and the International Narcotics Control Board's List of Psychotropic Substances under International Control, at http://www .incb.org/documents/Psychotropics/greenlist/Green_list_ENG _V17-06834.pdf.

TUBERCULOSIS

Healthcare providers can access professional consultation regarding tuberculosis evaluation and management from the CDC's TB Centers of Excellence for Training, Education, and Medical Consultation at https://www.cdc.gov/tb/education/tb_coe/default.htm.

Dive Medicine

If you are a scuba diver, membership in one or more of the following professional societies can help to keep you up to date regarding safe diving.

DIVE MEDICINE RESOURCES

Divers Alert Network
The Peter Bennett Center
6W Colony Pl.
Durham NC 27705-9815
tel. 919-684-2948
www.diversalertnetwork.org

Professional Association of Diving Instructors (PADI)
1251 East Dyer Road, #100
Santa Ana, CA 92705
tel. 714-540-7234
www.padi.com

Undersea and Hyperbaric Medical Society
10531 Metropolitan Ave.
Kensington MD 20895
tel. 301-942-2980
www.uhms.org

Conferences

If you are a nurse, doctor, pharmacist, dentist, nurse practitioner, physician's assistant, or other allied health professional, there are a number of excellent conferences on travel health:

- ISTM (www.istm.org) holds regular conferences, with all lectures in English, in a variety of countries.
- ASTMH (astmh.org) holds annual conferences at rotating sites within the US.
- The University of Washington hosts a two-and-a-half-day conference in Seattle, Washington, on travel medicine every two years (now on even years, to be offset from the ISTM Congresses). Information is available at: http://uwcme.org. (Full disclosure: I serve as chair of this course.)

GLOSSARY

antibody The molecule your body produces to fight a specific disease. The production of antibodies can be initiated by exposure to either a particular microorganism or a vaccine.

attenuated Weakened. Live vaccines are made with attenuated organisms. These are sufficiently similar to the wild type (i.e., variety in nature that can make you ill) to cause a protective antibody response but do not make you ill.

bactericidal Kills bacteria.

bacteriostatic Prevents bacteria from multiplying.

developing world A term that includes most of the world, excluding the US and Canada, Western Europe, Australia and New Zealand, Japan, and Singapore. Most countries in Africa, Latin America, and Asia are in the *developing world*. This term is falling out of favor; many people now refer to *low-* and *middle-income countries*, or the Global South.

diuretic Something that makes you urinate more.

edema Swelling or fluid leak. Edema of the ankles means swelling—that is, your ankles get a little fatter. In HAPE and HACE, edema refers to fluid leaking from blood vessels into the lungs or brain, respectively.

endemic Present in a particular place (e.g., malaria is endemic in the Amazon Basin).

epidemic An episode of more than usual or more than expected cases of an illness.

HIV Human immunodeficiency virus, the causative organism of AIDS (acquired immunodeficiency syndrome).

immune The state of being resistant to a disease.

immunosuppressed A lessened ability to fight disease. Examples of people who are immunosuppressed include those who are HIV-positive with low CD4 counts, people with malignancies, and those who take steroids chronically.

incubation period The duration between exposure to a microorganism and development of symptoms.

insect repellent Bugs whiff it, they don't like it, they fly in the other direction (e.g., DEET). Compare to *knockdown*.

jaundice Yellowing of the skin and sclerae (whites of the eyes); a symptom of liver disease, seen in diseases including hepatitis and yellow fever. The discoloration of the skin is more difficult to detect in dark-skinned people, but the change in color of the sclerae is evident in everyone.

knockdown A chemical that kills insects on contact (e.g., permethrin, which is applied to clothes).

pandemic A worldwide epidemic. Examples include the annual influenza epidemic seen in temperate latitudes and the current HIV pandemic.

pathogen A microorganism that can make you ill.

prophylactic Preventative.

sahel The border area between the Sahara Desert and tropical Africa.

South Asia Commonly used to refer to India, Pakistan, and Bangladesh; formerly termed the *Indian subcontinent*; more formally, also includes Nepal, Bhutan, Maldives, Sri Lanka, and Afghanistan.

STD Sexually transmitted disease, also known as STI: sexually transmitted infection.

subtropics The regions between the temperate regions and the tropics.

temperate regions Places farther from the equator than the subtropics (e.g., most of the US, most of Europe).

tropics Technically speaking, the area of the earth between 23°16' north and south latitudes (the Tropics of Cancer and Capricorn, respectively). More commonly used to refer to the warm regions near the equator.

tuk-tuk In Southeast Asia, taxis are most often *tuk-tuks*, which are motorcycles welded to a covered seat for two. In Peru these are known as *moto-taxis*.

VFR Acronym for "visiting friends and relatives," people born in low- and middle-income nations who move to a high-income nation, then return to their nation of birth to visit. This group is at higher-than-average risk for infectious diseases when they travel to low- and middle-income regions.

zoonosis Disease spread from animals to people.

INDEX

ABOUT THE AUTHOR

Christopher Sanford is a family medicine physician who specializes in travel and tropical medicine. Dr. Sanford is an associate professor in the Departments of Family Medicine and Global Health at the University of Washington (UW) in Seattle, Washington. He serves as director of the Travel Clinic, UW Neighborhood Northgate Clinic, and teaches in UW's Family Medicine Residency. He also serves as faculty for the Professional Diploma in Tropical Medicine and Hygiene (East African Partnership), an annual three-month course conducted in Uganda and Tanzania. He is lead editor of *Travel and Tropical Medicine Manual*, 5th edition, and writes regularly on travel and tropical medicine for a number of publications, including the *Merck Manual* (both professional and home editions).

Dr. Sanford earned a master of public health degree at the Harvard School of Public Health; a diploma in tropical medicine and hygiene from Universidad Peruana Cayetano Heredia and the Gorgas Memorial Institute of Tropical and Preventative Medicine in Lima, Peru; an MD from the University of California, San Diego; a BA in psychology from the University of California, Santa Barbara; and no degree from El Camino College in Torrance, California, despite two and a half years of classes with excellent teachers. He completed a residency in family medicine at San Jose Medical Center/Stanford University (now San Jose–O'Connor Hospital Family Medicine Residency). He has been awarded a Certificate of Knowledge in Clinical Tropical Medicine and Travelers' Health from the American Society of Tropical Medicine and Hygiene. He is board certified in Family Medicine.

In addition to teaching each year in Uganda, Dr. Sanford enjoys travel to pretty much everywhere on the planet. He lives in Seattle with his wife and two sons.